e-Pathways

Computers and the patient's journey through care

Edited by

Kathryn de Luc MSc, MBA, PhD

Healthcare Research Consultant

and

Julian Todd MSc

Health Systems Strategy Manager
Dudley Group of Hospitals NHS Trust

Foreword by

JA Muir Gray

Director
National electronic Library for Health

Radcliffe Medical Press

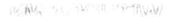

Radcliffe Medical Press Ltd
18 Marcham Road
Abingdon
Oxon OX14 1AA
United Kingdom

www.radcliffe-oxford.com
The Radcliffe Medical Press electronic catalogue and online ordering facility.
Direct sales to anywhere in the world.

£28.23

British Library Cataloguing in Publication Data

A catalogue record for this book is available from the British Library.

ISBN 1 85775 903 6

Typeset by Joshua Associates Ltd, Oxford
Printed and bound by TJ International Ltd, Padstow, Cornwall

Contents

Foreword   iv
Preface   vi
List of contributors   xv
Acknowledgements   xvii

1   Introduction
    Kathryn de Luc and Julian Todd   1

PART ONE   15

2   Knowledge management (clinical evidence)
    Bertha Yuen Man Low and Pam Prior   17

3   Care pathway development
    Chris Homer and Linda Dunn   45

4   Building a computerised care pathway: practical lessons
    Margaret Craddock   81

PART TWO   107

5   A systems view of care pathways
    Julian Todd   109

6   Developing e-pathway standards
    Ruth Page and Ian Herbert   155

7   A way forward?
    Kathryn de Luc and Julian Todd   183

Care pathway related websites   199

Glossary   213
Index   223

Foreword

The most important question for any organisation to address in the 21st century is the function of the human being. Bill Gates, who first asked this question, was thinking about banks and travel agents when he posed it, but it is just as relevant to healthcare. Human beings have strengths and weaknesses and we now know that human beings are poor at remembering things, get bored with routine tasks, and like to be creative. The type of education we give healthcare professionals, while rightly emphasising that each individual is unique, also suggests that each healthcare problem has a unique scientific solution.

Clinical decisions have three main inputs – scientific evidence, the condition of the particular patient, and the patient's values. We now have plenty of evidence that computers are much better than human beings at remembering evidence and presenting it when it is needed in the course of a patient's care. Human beings, if properly taught, are much better at relating the evidence to the individual patient's condition and helping the patient reflect on the options that face them, although computers can help with the latter task. Care pathways help clinicians carry out the human side of the task well by removing the need for them to remember all the routine aspects of care and thus preventing the errors that occur from slips and omissions. Either on paper or on a computer screen, the care pathway can contribute to better quality healthcare and clinical practice.

I look forward to a day when the letter that invites me to hospital also contains the first steps of the care pathway – for example, advising me to stop smoking if I am coming for an operation, and telling me where I can get help. I look forward to the day when I arrive at the hospital and by the time they have typed in 'Muir', not a particularly common name in Oxford, up will pop for the clinician and for me any evidence that has been produced since I was last at the hospital. I look forward to a day on which the clinician can spend time discussing the likelihood of being helped or the likelihood of being harmed by various interventions, safe in the knowledge that the clinician's memory has not been the only tool that has led them to remember that I should be offered these options.

The pathways will increase and not decrease the human side of healthcare and we welcome their prominent place in the National electronic Library for Health.

This excellent book provides both a justification for, and an introduction to, this revolutionary concept which was at one time seen as the preserve of nurses but which should permeate the whole of healthcare.

JA Muir Gray CBE, DSc, MD, FRCP, FRCPSGlas
Director
National electronic Library for Health
June 2003

Preface

Key points

- Much of the development of care pathways in the UK is fragmented with patchy take-up and use of the concept.

- Great duplication of effort in care pathway development is occurring across the UK.

- The full potential of care pathways as a quality improvement technique is not being realised, neither in paper nor electronic form.

Why we wrote this book

The current approach to care pathway development in the United Kingdom (UK) can be summarised as 'reinventing wheels on an industrial scale'. A search on the current care pathway database on the National electronic Library for Health (NeLH) demonstrates the extent to which there has been duplication of pathway development effort at local healthcare provider level. For example, fractured neck of femur care pathways are listed by over 60 different National Health Service (NHS) organisations. Yet at the same time the number of organisations that have large numbers of care pathways in use is relatively small in the UK. Scrivener (2000)[1] points out that the NeLH database shows that the range of pathways per organisation is between one and 141 and the mode, i.e.

the most frequently occurring number per organisation, is only two. So we have the paradox of a large amount of replication of effort occurring for certain conditions/diseases but only patchy take-up of the concept across individual healthcare organisations.

The editors of this book consider this to be a fundamental problem of fragmentation – the disjointed and *ad hoc* way in which care pathways are being developed does not present a full and coherent picture of their possibilities. As a result, we believe the full potential of care pathways as a quality improvement technique is not being realised.

Within UK healthcare organisations, care pathways as a concept are probably at a critical point in their development. The situation has moved a long way from the early 1990s when small clinical teams working in a hospital setting and using a 'bottom-up' approach decided to develop a care pathway for a particular elective surgical procedure, often in response to a particular clinical problem. Nowadays, care pathways are often extended out of the hospital environment to cover patient/client journeys that cross primary and secondary care, or to cover services in mental health and learning disabilities and to involve other agencies, including ambulance services, social services and education.

Healthcare organisations are asking: what percentage of patients can we cover with care pathways? Is the percentage large enough to allow us to use the tool to plan the delivery of services on a strategic, community-wide basis? Can a healthcare organisation use the tool to assist with planning new healthcare building projects, or to commission services on the basis of care pathways?

The UK information strategy for the modern NHS 1998–2005 (1998)[2] required that acute trusts implement care pathways within clinical computer systems – a trend which is reflected in other countries. While the details of implementation have been left to local interpretation, it is clear that computerisation of care pathways offers significant opportunities and challenges. How should care pathways be developed and structured so they can be implemented in computerised work-flow systems?

Such questions take care pathways into another order of magnitude from the committed clinical team developing a single care pathway. If care pathways are to adopt this wider role then we argue that a more systemic and systematic approach to the development of care pathways is needed – we need to be developing and sharing '*e-pathways*'.

This book considers definitions of, and standards for, care pathways in some detail because we believe that the lack of comprehensive, agreed definitions is a fundamental problem. Care pathways sit at the centre of many agendas and concepts, which goes part way to explaining why different people and groups have different ideas of what care pathways are and what they can do.

Figure 1 shows a map of some of the relevant concepts and how they interrelate. This shows the complexity of the care pathways topic area. The diagram is not intended as a definitive statement, but as a graphical aid to thinking about this complexity. The central themes of the book are indicated by the darker shaded ovals – the **patient's journey** through the health/social care system is based on one or more **care pathways**, with all the detail of both planned and actual care being recorded in one or more **clinical computer systems**.

The pale shaded ovals in Figure 1 represent additional core topics of the book, which, we argue, need to be managed in a structured way if the potential benefits of computerisation are to be realised. The remaining topics shown indicate some of the wide range of related issues. By following the concepts and relationship arrows we can start to map at a high level the influence which care pathways can have on how healthcare is delivered. For example, a **care pathway** *is based on* **evidence,** *which facilitates* **decision support**, *which supports* **evidence-based practice**, *which supports* **clinical governance.**

The prospect of computerising care pathways increases both the complexity and the challenges of their development and implementation. Policy makers and many clinical and management staff at local level clearly believe that it is worth tackling this challenge. Both the editors and chapter authors strongly support this view and we hope this book will help.

The purpose of this book

The purpose of this book is threefold:

- to discuss how one might develop a more systematic approach to care pathway development
- to explore the potential for information technology (IT) and systems thinking in the further development and implementation of care pathways
- to stimulate debate, discussion and critique about the function and form of e-pathways.

Inevitably this book will represent a 'snapshot' of the thinking in 2002 of some of the various contributors who are working within this field. Over time, such thinking will evolve, develop and change. Our aim in producing this book has been to provide the opportunity and mechanism to debate the future function and role of e-pathways. This is something we feel rarely happens in the care pathway literature at the moment.

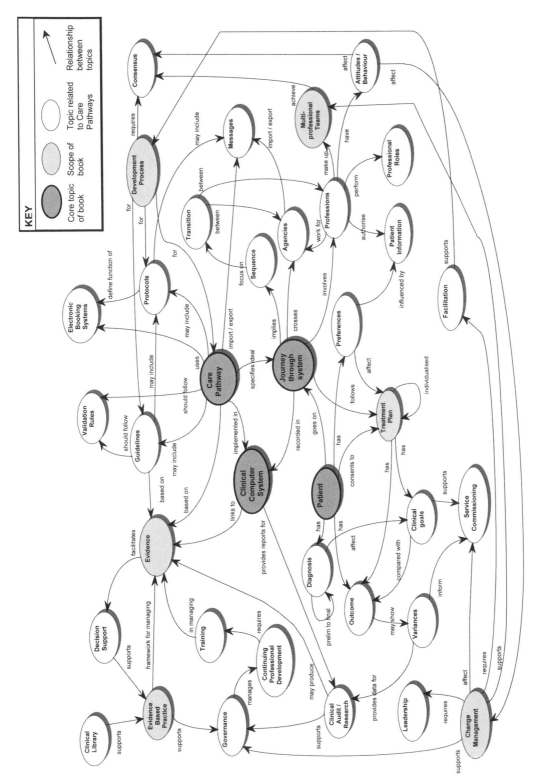

Figure 1 Care pathway concept map.

For whom is this book written?

This book is intended mainly for those who already have a working knowledge of care pathways. It is not a book for care pathway beginners. If you are just learning about care pathways then we would recommend you first read one or more of the introductory books on the subject, including de Luc (2000)[3] Johnson (1997),[4] Middleton and Roberts (2000),[5] Zander (1995)[6] and Dykes and Wheeler (1997),[7] or look at the 'general information on care pathways' websites listed at the end of the book.

This book is written for a wide range of people who will have different perspectives and interests in care pathways. It will be relevant to:

- people from a clinical background who have had some experience of working with pathways either in their development or in using them in clinical practice
- healthcare management staff who are interested in exploring the potential of care pathways for the strategic development of their organisations
- Information technology specialists who want to understand how the IT tools and approaches familiar to them can be harnessed and used within a care pathway context.

Our aim is to draw together these different perspectives and explore the knowledge and expertise which exists, but which we believe has yet to be fully utilised within the context of e-pathways.

How to use this book

This book is in two parts. In Part One, Chapters 2, 3 and 4 take as their main theme three of the main current challenges (or limitations) for care pathway developers. These limitations are:

- clinical evidence management for care pathways at local, national and international levels
- individual pathway development, implementation and maintenance in multi-professional, multi-agency teams
- implementing care pathways in clinical computer systems.

In Part One we highlight where IT-based approaches can help what could be called 'conventional' approaches to the development and implementation of care pathways, which have so far made little use of IT. Every attempt has been made to cover this material in non-technical language.

In Part Two, Chapters 5 and 6 introduce various systems concepts and techniques which address two further limitations of conventional approaches. These limitations are:

- how to support whole-community organisational change management using care pathways
- lack of clarity of concepts and definitions for care pathways and related topics which are universally understood and accepted and required for effective, widespread computerisation.

Of necessity, Chapters 5 and 6 contain more technical material than Part One, so a summary of the main points is provided on p. 107 at the beginning of Part Two.

A brief overview of the content of all the chapters is provided below to help direct the reader.

Part One

- Chapter 1: **Introduction**. This chapter identifies some of the limitations with care pathways as they are being conceptualised and developed, and discusses the ramifications of the conventional approach. These issues provide the framework for the focus of each of the following chapters.
- Chapter 2: **Knowledge management (clinical evidence)**. This chapter illustrates how knowledge management can be used to underpin the clinical evidence contained within care pathways and provides a framework for doing so.
- Chapter 3: **Care pathway development**. This chapter focuses on the role of care pathways as a change management tool. It concentrates on the human aspects of pathway development, i.e. the individuals involved in pathway development, and provides some guidance on the key issues to be considered.
- Chapter 4: **Building a computerised care pathway – practical lessons**. This chapter describes one trust's experiences with trying to computerise a care pathway in stroke services as part of its clinical computer system development.

Part Two

- Chapter 5: **A systems view of care pathways**. This chapter explores the potential for systems thinking, process modelling and process redesign within the context of care pathways. Example case studies are used to illustrate how different aspects of systems thinking can help in the development and implementation of pathways at a whole-community level.

- Chapter 6: **Developing e-pathway standards**. This chapter explores the relationship between similar but distinct concepts from care pathways, including guidelines, protocols etc., then describes recent work on modelling these concepts and relationships to provide definitions which could become national standards.
- Chapter 7: **A way forward?** This chapter summarises the key arguments running through this book and makes some suggestions as to the way the ideas might be taken forward within a systems framework.

At the end of the book is a list of websites related to care pathways. The purpose of this list is to provide a concise reference to information that is available on the web which relates specifically to care pathways. Please note that throughout this book reference is made to many other relevant websites, but which do not necessarily focus specifically on the care pathway topic.

Finally, a glossary of terms has been included for two reasons. Firstly, successful development, implementation and maintenance of e-pathways depend on a wider knowledge base and team membership than is associated with conventional care pathways. Secondly, this book is aimed at a wider range of readers than most care pathway literature.

How to use the CD

Accompanying this book is a CD containing supplementary information. Our objectives for including the CD are to:

- provide additional material on specific topics, so that the main book remains accessible to as wide a range of readers as possible
- provide direct links both to Internet resources cited in the text and to additional sites of general interest
- save download time by providing some of the larger files on the CD.

Readers should please note:

- Although the editors and authors have made all reasonable efforts to check that hyperlinks and downloaded documents are accurate and up to date, this cannot be guaranteed and the CD is provided 'as is'.
- Internet based material changes rapidly, so the information on the CD will be more up to date than that printed in the book, because of the different production timescales.
- CD material is not covered by the copyright restrictions of the book. The editors and authors of this book have obtained papers and other

material from public websites or with the authors' permission. Reuse of the information on the CD is governed by the copyright restrictions on the original sources – that is, inclusion on the CD does not indicate that material is copyright-free. Readers should consult the original source of each document for further details, if required.

The CD is structured as a self-contained 'website'. It should run automatically on any PC running *Microsoft Windows 95* or later and web browser software such as *Microsoft Internet Explorer version 5*, or *Netscape Navigator version 4*, or above. If the CD home page does not load automatically, it can be launched manually by opening the file 'index.htm' in the top-level directory of the CD, using your web browser 'File Open' command. No direct support for Apple Macintosh computers is provided.*

From the CD home page you will be able to navigate to:

- chapter-by-chapter summaries, plus tables of hyperlinks relevant to each chapter. These include websites and files on the CD in either HTML or Adobe Acrobat (pdf) format. To view the latter, you will require the free Adobe Acrobat reader. A link to the Adobe website to download the latest version is also included, if required
- a separate section provided by Popkin Software & Systems Ltd, which includes a 30-day evaluation copy of their *Systems Architect* systems modelling software, plus an example 'encyclopaedia' from the care pathway modelling described in Chapter 5
- an updated copy of the list of care pathway related websites, with direct hyperlinks to these resources.

Kathryn de Luc
Julian Todd
June 2003

References

1   Scrivener R (2002) Personal communication.
2   NHS Executive (1998) *Information for Health: an information strategy for the modern NHS 1998–2005*. Department of Health, London.
3   de Luc K (2000) *Developing Care Pathways: the handbook and the tool kit*. Radcliffe Medical Press, Oxford.

---

* The behaviour of the CD and its contents will depend on many local factors beyond the control of the editors, Radcliffe Medical Press and Popkin Software & Systems Ltd. We regret that we cannot provide technical support or any warranty.

4   Johnson S (1997) *Pathways of Care*. Blackwell Science, Oxford.
5   Middleton S and Roberts A (2000) *Integrated Care Pathways: a practical approach to implementation*. Butterworth-Heinemann, Oxford.
6   Zander K (ed.) (1995) *Managing Outcomes through Collaborative Care: the application of care mapping and case management*. American Hospital Publishing, Inc., USA.
7   Dykes P and Wheeler K (1997) *Planning, Implementing and Evaluating Critical Pathways*. Springer Publishing, New York.

Kathryn de Luc is now living and working in New Zealand. Her email address is kathydeluc@snap.net.nz.

The editors would encourage all readers interested in the further development of e-pathways to sample the online communities at www.venturetc.com/discussion_forum.asp and www.smartgroups.com/groups/clinicalpathways.

List of contributors

Our thanks go to those who have contributed chapters and case study material to this book.

Chapter authors

Chapter 2: Bertha Yuen Man Low and Pam Prior, West Midlands Regional Library Unit.

Chapter 3: Chris Homer and Linda Dunn, Partnership for Developing Quality, West Midlands Region.

Chapter 4: Margaret Craddock, Walsall Integrated Stroke Service, Walsall Primary Care Trust.

Chapter 6: Ruth Page and Ian Herbert, NHS Information Authority.

Contributors of case study and other materials used in the book and CD

- Lisa Day, Process Mapping Co-ordinator, West Sussex Shared Services Consortium for the example of process mapping contained within Chapter 5.
- Sarah Ives and Sally Reid, Redesign and Development Leads, Oxfordshire Patient Access Improvement Team (host organisation – Oxford Radcliffe Hospitals Trust) for the example of applying the theory of constraints contained within Chapter 5.

- Chris Taylor, Retired Clinical Director, A&E, Queen Mary's Hospital, Sidcup for the FlowForma clinical guidelines information contained within Chapter 5.
- Sarah Caldicott, Integrated Care Pathway Co-ordinator, Hereford Acute Hospitals; Sandi Kirkham, Principal Lecturer, School of Computing, University of Central England in Birmingham and Helen Sudlow, Clinical Governance Co-ordinator, Herefordshire Primary Care Trust for their example of applying the soft systems methodology (SSM) approach to care pathways contained within Chapter 5.
- Paul Newrick, Consultant Diabetologist, Worcestershire Acute Hospitals NHS Trust for use of the diabetic ketoacidosis care pathway used to illustrate the systems models contained within Chapters 5 and 6.
- Ross Scrivener, Information Manager, Quality Improvement Programme, Royal College of Nursing for information on care pathway websites.
- Kris Vanhaecht, Clinical Pathway Network Co-ordinator, The Belgium–Dutch Clinical Pathway Network for information on care pathway websites.
- Alan Fisher, Integrated Care Pathway Facilitator, Clinical Audit Resource Centre, Western General Hospital, Edinburgh for information on care pathway websites.
- Barbara Bolton, Clinical Librarian, Dudley Group of Hospitals NHS Trust for websites contained within Chapter 2.
- Orion Systems New Zealand Ltd for illustrations of the computerised stroke care pathway contained within Chapter 4.

Acknowledgements

This book was conceived as a result of work on the computerisation of care pathways that took place between 2000 and 2002 in the West Midlands Region. The Partnership for Developing Quality (PDQ) and the Regional Information Strategy Board supported a group of interested healthcare workers from various organisations across the region and the NHS Information Authority to form an e-pathways working group. This group commissioned two pieces of work, namely Flower et al. (2001)[1] and Oswald (2001),[2] and also held a regional conference on the e-pathways topic in April 2001.

Over the past two years the e-pathways work has led the editors of this book to many contacts and networks across the UK and internationally where like-minded thinking and interest in the topic is developing. Our thanks go to all those people with whom we have been in contact – the discussions and lively debates that we had during this time have informed much of the thinking that is reflected in this book. All the individuals whom we have been in contact with are too numerous to name here but we would like to thank in particular:

- Linda Dunn, Professional Development Co-ordinator, Partnership for Developing Quality – West Midlands
- Judith Le Maistre, former Director of Health Informatics, Herefordshire Health Service
- Paul Shobrook, former Deputy Regional Head of Information, West Midlands Region
- The Partnership for Developing Quality and the Regional Information Strategy Steering Group (for allocation of project funding and staff time).

People who contributed to the e-pathways group included: Anne Brice; Charles Bruce; Jessica Flower; Paul Frosdick; Nick Gaunt; David Jones;

Maxine Jones; Bala Kainth; Louise MacPherson; Shiv Naraynen; Malcolm Oswald; David Rodrick; Susan Short; John Thornbury; Pat Williams.

The editors would also like to thank the following people and organisations that have helped with this book:

- Joyce Smith, Dudley Group of Hospitals for administrative support
- Technical and marketing staff at Popkin Software & Systems Ltd for supporting the CD that accompanies this book
- Claire Whittle, Lecturer in Nursing, the School of Health Sciences, University of Birmingham for comments on the manuscript
- Dr Clive Leyland, Chairman, IT Programme Board, Dudley Group of Hospitals for comments on the manuscript.

References

1 Flower J, Geernaert M and Hartsorn A (2001) *Review of issues and options for creating, storing and using electronic care pathways across the NHS*. BBD Consultancy Services, Lichfield. *See* CD.
2 Oswald M (2001) *West Midlands Regional e-Pathways Project Final Report: exploring the usefulness of the healthcare model in developing integrated care pathways*. West Midlands Region, Birmingham. Unpublished.

Dedication

This book is dedicated to Stafford Beer, a leading exponent of the application of systems thinking to organisations, who died shortly before this book was finished.

Stafford Beer founded the systems discipline of Management Cybernetics, or 'the science of effective organisation'. Despite (or perhaps because of) his background in wartime operations research, he consistently applied his innovative and radical ideas about how organisations actually work and could work better in ways which promoted the greatest possible autonomy, at the lowest possible level, throughout an organisation. We think he would have immediately recognised and supported the goals and methods of multidisciplinary care pathway teams. He pioneered the application of computing, telecommunications and what would nowadays be called 'knowledge management' to large, complex organisations 30 years ago, and so we think he would have also applauded the concept of e-pathways.

He wrote many books and papers, but a quote will give a flavour of his approach to participative change management:

> 'Every time we hear that a proposal will destroy society as we know it, we should have the courage to say "Thank God; at last."'

Stafford Beer
25 September 1926–23 August 2002

1

Introduction

Kathryn de Luc and Julian Todd

Key points

- There are important limitations with care pathways as they are currently conceived in a paper-based format.

- The limitations identified are:
  - the need for ongoing clinical evidence management within care pathways
  - the development, implementation and maintenance of care pathways
  - the obstacles to moving away from paper-based care pathways and embedding them in clinical computer systems
  - achieving a whole-community organisational change management approach for care pathways
  - the lack of clarity of the concept and definitions which are universally understood and accepted.

Ethos of care pathways

Currie and Harvey (2000)[1] make the point that care pathways (also called critical paths, clinical pathways, care tracks, integrated care pathways [ICPs], care maps) are being introduced in many healthcare systems around the world with the aim of improving the quality of healthcare. Harkleroad *et al.* (2000)[2] point out that the concept of care pathways borrows much from the theories of continuous quality improvement

(CQI), and as Johnson (1997)[3] argues, in order for a CQI programme to be successful it is essential for all staff who are involved in seeing patients to receive feedback on the analyses of care so that they can see if they are performing against expected standards and guidelines and how they might continue to improve. Ahgren (2001)[4] argues that over the past two decades there has been an acceleration of sub-specialisation in healthcare as medical science and technology have progressed. This has led to a fragmentation of the healthcare system, making collaboration and communication between healthcare personnel very difficult when viewed from the horizontal perspective of the patient's journey. The need to develop seamless services tailored to patients' needs rather than how the healthcare organisations are structured has been recognised in *The NHS Plan* (2000),[5] and various NHS National Service Frameworks (NSFs) (2000)[6] (2001),[7] which set standards of healthcare across the NHS. In the United States (US) this requirement to develop patient-focused, seamless care is referred to as an integrated delivery system.

There is no single agreed definition of a care pathway. It is a complex and multifaceted concept. Pearson *et al.* (1995)[8] define a care pathway as 'a management plan that displays goals for patients and provides the sequence and timing of actions necessary to achieve these goals with optimal efficiency'. Middleton and Roberts (2000)[9] define the concept as 'an outline or plan of anticipated clinical practice for a group of patients (client group) with a particular diagnosis or set of symptoms. It provides a multidisciplinary template of the plan of care, leading each patient towards a desired objective.' Both of these definitions highlight the planning function of care pathways. However, in our view neither of these definitions capture the dynamic and developmental nature of care pathways. It has been highlighted by de Luc (2000)[10] that the care pathway concept consists of both a process (of development and continuing maintenance) and a set of operational products (including the process work-flow or process map, clinical documentation and information for reviewing care and the use of resources on an ongoing basis). This latter information is produced mainly from variance (or exception) reporting, where staff record any variations from the care pathway for individual patients.

The benefits listed by advocates of care pathways include:

- greater consistency in practice
- improved continuity of care
- monitored standards of care
- improved clinical documentation
- the implementation of evidence-based practice
- the delivery of care which is patient-focused and designed around the patient's/user's requirements rather than the organisation.

Flower *et al.* (2001)[11] highlight how a care pathway focuses on linking evidence and guidance to a set of care processes and continually evaluating them. For each process a linking of a number of elements needs to be supported, including:

- the care objectives and goals associated with the process
- a detailed description of the healthcare activities associated with the process
- access to clinical guidance to evaluate efficacious interventions (decision support information)
- facilities to record and monitor the care and administrative actions taken
- facilities to control and report on activities that are at variance to the planned care pathway.

The concept of care pathways has not escaped criticism and several barriers to their development have been identified. These include:

- the need to ensure that all disciplines involved in patient care will engage in the development of care pathways and will change their behaviour/clinical practice as required
- lack of guidance on the methodology for development and implementation
- the inflexibility of care pathway paper documentation
- the amount of resources and time required to both develop and maintain effective and efficient care pathways
- the sheer size of the task in developing care pathways to cover all care processes.

The next section of this chapter considers some of the limitations outlined by critics of the concept of care pathways as they are currently perceived and asks the question: can the greater use of IT and the computerisation of care pathways help with some of these issues?

Limitations of care pathways

We have identified five broad limitations with care pathways in their current state of development where we believe significant improvement can be made by the use of IT and systems thinking. These limitations are:

1 the need for ongoing clinical evidence management within care pathways
2 the development, implementation and maintenance of care pathways

3 the obstacles to moving away from paper-based care pathways and embedding them in clinical computer systems

4 achieving a whole-community organisational change management approach for care pathways

5 the lack of clarity of the concept and definitions which are universally understood and accepted.

Limitation 1: The need for ongoing clinical evidence management within care pathways

As Currie and Harvey (2000)[1] pointed out, one of the fundamental objectives of care pathways is to support evidence-based practice, or if the evidence base is lacking, to support structured clinical audit in monitoring outcomes and variations. This information helps to achieve improved practice through the principle of continuous quality improvement.

It has been well documented that variation in clinical practice continues even when guidelines based on reputable evidence exists. The need for increased standardisation of clinical decision making has been recognised by a number of authors – Morris (2000),[12] Grol and Grimshaw (1999),[13] Gross and Romano (2001),[14] NHS Centre for Reviews and Dissemination (1999).[15] Care pathways (together with guidelines and protocols) attempt to introduce greater standardisation and to reduce the unnecessary variations in practice.

However, to fulfil this role reliably one has to ensure that the care pathway is always up to date, is based on the latest evidence and that the information contained within it (and on which clinical staff decide treatment options for individual patients) is readily accessible at the interaction with the patient. Currently, many care pathways do not provide explicit references to their evidence nor do they indicate how they have used the evidence in developing the content of the care pathway.

The problem of the sheer volume of, and rate of increase in, clinical evidence being too great for any practising clinician to handle has been recognised. Morris (2000)[12] argues that excess information in complex clinical environments increases the likelihood of clinical errors. Front-line clinicians (and managers) who are trying to improve service quality need high-quality information, which must be relevant, reliable, timely and easily accessible. Although there are structured methods for assessing evidence together with standards for representing bibliographic citations, these are rarely incorporated into a care pathway. We believe that organisations need to have in place a system for ensuring that the content of all their care pathways is reviewed and updated regularly (minimum annually) by reference to the latest clinical evidence. Otherwise care pathways can easily become obsolete and stagnant. Organisations need to ensure that there are the skills in, and time for, searching and appraising evidence, and for clinical staff to update their knowledge of the literature. Such knowledge management is clearly a demanding, long-term objective. It requires improved ways of structuring and locating relevant information, specialists to sift and moderate evidence for specific constituencies and easy-to-use retrieval systems. We would argue it is an inordinate waste of everyone's time to be replicating this effort in every healthcare organisation.

Chapter 2 addresses this issue of knowledge management within the context of care pathways. It suggests a methodology for assembling this knowledge base. It also includes a case study about maintaining the evidence base for a chest pain and myocardial infarction care pathway at national level.

Limitation 2: The development, implementation and maintenance of care pathways

Campbell *et al.* (1998),[16] Layton *et al.* (1998)[17] and Togno-Armanasco *et al.* (1993)[18] all make the point that care pathways are time-consuming to construct. They require effort and commitment from the clinical team developing them, together with top-down support from the organisation(s) in which the care pathway is being developed. As March *et al.* (2000)[19] point out, this can make their development expensive in use of staff, which is a barrier to development.

De Luc (2002)[20] has identified ten steps to the development of individual care pathways. These are listed below:

Planning stage
 1 Project plan the development of individual care pathways.
 2 Obtain information on patients'/users' views, critical incident/near misses, the clinical evidence/guidelines, relevant legislation, activity and access information and sample pathways from other organisations.

Development stage
 3 Scope the care pathway (identify the beginning and end points) and identify objectives and measurable goals.
 4 Process map and redesign the services.
 5 Design the care pathway documentation.

Implementation stage
 6 Plan for the changes in process (undertake gap analysis).
 7 Train the staff to use the care pathway.

8 Test (or pilot) the care pathway.
9 Sign off the care pathway (gain approval for use within the organisation).
10 Ensure ongoing maintenance and updating of the care pathway based on analysis of the variances and standards of care achieved.

Care pathway development requires facilitation, discussion and debate to decide content. In a sense care pathways are never finished as they require regular updates in the light of new information. The cyclical nature of the development process is illustrated in Figure 1.1.

Recent NHS initiatives have encouraged local communities to restructure clinical services in terms of the patient journey and process/work-flow, but local teams are essentially still left to their own devices in terms of skills, tools and models to use. Given the complexity of the task of development of a single care pathway, organisations need to plan for several meetings per pathway. If you extend this estimate to calculate the resources needed to develop care pathways across the entire NHS for all

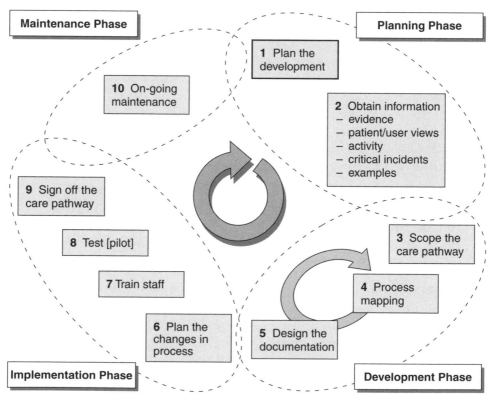

Figure 1.1 Ten steps to developing a care pathway.

the conditions possible, it seems likely that you are describing a multimillion pound use of resource.

The question must be asked: would the greater sharing of care pathways and lessons learnt in developing them make it easier and quicker to develop one's own care pathway? Care pathways are essentially a change management tool and a key consideration for their successful development and implementation highlighted in the ten-step guide is the nature of the development process. There needs to be a sense of involvement and ownership, felt by the various constituencies who will make the pathway work in practice. Whilst we would not advocate an attempt to transfer any single care pathway from one site to another (this is unlikely to be successful), we believe that there needs to be a structuring and dissemination of 'how to' knowledge about care pathways which can support their development along with easy access to other organisations' care pathways to review and compare.

Chapter 3 discusses many of these 'how to' issues and lists many further sources of information on the subject.

Limitation 3: The obstacles to moving away from paper-based care pathways and embedding them in clinical computer systems

One objective of care pathways is to improve the quality of clinical documentation. The Clinical Systems Group (1998)[21] highlighted the research that showed poor communications and poor documentation processes exacerbate fragmentation of care across a range of professional groups. Various authors, including the Council of International Hospitals (1995),[22] Lau et al. (1996)[23] and Hotchkiss (1997),[24] have argued that care pathways provide benefits in the following areas relating to clinical documentation:

- streamlining clinical documentation
- improving the completeness, legibility and accuracy of clinical documentation
- improving communication between members of the clinical team in the management of patients
- using the documentation to prompt or aid clinical decision making
- providing a structured audit tool to review standards of care and variances.

Currently, care pathways are predominantly text based and deployed as document sets. As Currie and Scrivener (in press)[25] point out, within the UK only a minority of pathways have been embedded in proprietary work-flow systems, or have had their logic and forms coupled to computer software. However, paper-based care pathways do have limitations. Chu (2001)[26] goes as far as to say that the paper tool has failed to function effectively as a product quality assurance instrument. Some of the limitations of paper-based care pathways include:

- **The length and amount of detail contained within a paper care pathway**. Care pathways that contain a lot of detail can become cumbersome and unwieldy. Conversely, documents that are kept short and concise lose some of the important clinical detail needed to prompt staff in decision making.
- **The difficulty in individualising patient care whilst standardising clinical decision making**. Morris (2000),[12] for example, criticises care pathways because they are time-driven decision support tools which, he argues, are unable to deliver individualised, patient-specific treatment. The paper care pathway template is fixed and, whilst one can individualise care through the use of exception reporting or the recording of individual variances, the rigidity of the paper document makes this more difficult. Similarly, paper care pathways do not deal well with the concept of a 'floating activity' that can be done when certain criteria are met rather than at a certain time.
- **The difficulty of dealing with complexity and unpredictability in patients with multi-problems/co-morbidities**. This is similar in nature to the problem of individualising care using paper care pathways but constitutes a larger and more fundamental problem. Whilst strategies for dealing with this problem have been devised in paper formats with, for example, 'co-pathways' advocated by Dykes (1998)[27] – these can be inserted into the main care pathway – there still remains a lack of flexibility to deal with this problem in paper format.
- **The storage of the paper documentation whilst in use and once completed.** The Council of International Hospitals report on the case study at the Central Middlesex Hospital (1995)[22] points out that whilst seemingly a minor issue, this can prove the most difficult to address. Paper documentation can only be at one location at any one time, yet it is common for more than one member of the clinical team to need the patient record simultaneously and particularly so when the care pathway crosses organisational boundaries. In addition, once the care pathway is completed, the issue of ownership and storage of the documentation can cause tension as the various organisations need to meet their operational requirements and legal obligations.
- **The manual analysis of the data (including variances) collected from using the care pathway**. Care pathways collect a large amount of data which needs to be analysed and evaluated both for the provision of

individual patient care (real-time analysis) and retrospectively, when reviewing the last, say, 50–100 care pathway documents. All of this information needs to be presented to the clinical staff using the care pathways so that they can use it to review the care being delivered and identify areas for change and improvement. If analysed regularly, Jones *et al.* (1999)[28] argue that the information can also be utilised in the planning of services, reviewing the use of resources and facilities and in the costing of care.

The above points will be familiar to anyone who has been involved in the design and use of clinical documentation to support a care pathway. However, perhaps the biggest and most significant disadvantage of putting a care pathway into a paper format is that this medium cannot show the structure, process steps and decision trees within the pathway, i.e. the pathway is stored/presented as essentially a list, with:

- no means of zooming in and out of detail
- no means of placing the pathway process flow within a broader organisational context (e.g. the reform of outpatient services)
- no easy means of sharing common functions across different pathways
- no easy means of translating from paper-based to clinical computer system-based deployment
- no easy means of cataloguing the pathway and its constituent parts.

We consider that a clinical computer system could make implementation of care pathways easier in several ways, namely:

- improved data collection – management by exception and rapid data entry
- online access to guidelines/evidence/technical information
- decision support environment
- grouped functions – test sets, drug regimens and packages of care can be ordered in one operation, thus saving time and reducing errors
- facilitation of clinical audit through patient-based data and clinical coding/terming
- improved data quality through elimination of duplication of information and handwritten notes
- flexibility – elements can be added to or deleted from a care pathway to create a care plan tailored to the patient, without loss of data quality for the individual patient episode
- multiple staff can view the clinical record from different locations simultaneously
- individualisation of the 'view' of the clinical record for different staff or staff groups so that it becomes easier to find relevant information.

Chapter 4 describes one health community's experience with computerising a stroke care pathway and reinforces many of the advantages listed above.

Despite the fact that care pathways and clinical computer systems are mutually supportive, the recent care pathways survey reported by Currie and Scrivener (in press)[25] has indicated that implementation of care pathways in EPR systems is still a distant prospect for most sites. We believe that progress towards this target would be much quicker if we began to look at the concept of care pathways in a more structured and systematic way and shared the lessons learnt.

Limitation 4: Achieving a whole-community organisational change management approach for care pathways

Part of the reason that so much of the material relevant to care pathways is fragmented is because the subject area is very wide. The concept map included within the preface to this book has already illustrated this point. To achieve successful care pathway development and implementation across a whole organisation or health community, we need to draw upon information relating to clinical staff and how they integrate the latest clinical evidence, how they operate as a clinical team, their professional roles and how they plan, deliver and record clinical care. We also need information from a management perspective in terms of managing change, leadership, and the strategic role of the organisation in supporting clinical staff to develop, implement and maintain their care pathways. Information is also required from an IT and systems thinking perspective in terms of modelling services, process redesign, decision support systems, computerised record keeping and document control systems (including version controls and changes in content).

Chapter 5 explores the application of systems thinking, modelling and redesign to care pathways to see if this approach can help with the achievement of whole-community/organisational change management.

Limitation 5: The lack of clarity of the concept and definitions which are universally understood and accepted

Several writers, including Morris (2000),[12] Every *et al.* (2000)[29] and Trowbridge and Weingarten (2001),[30] have highlighted the confusion between the different but similar concepts of clinical guidelines, protocols and care pathways. This confusion is well illustrated by the use of the term 'pathway' in some of the National Service Framework documents in the UK. Johnson (2001)[31] points out that the name is used to describe essentially different tools, i.e. a simple process map to illustrate patient flows for a particular disease group through the healthcare system, or a document that replaces the individual patient record. Consequently, no agreed set of national definitions and standards exists of the functional elements (objects) that comprise the building blocks of a care pathway. There is also a wide variety of formats for pathway modelling and documentation.

So what is the relationship between the concepts of guidelines, protocols and care pathways? Is one a subset of another? Trowbridge and Weingarten (2001)[30] amongst others have tried to clarify some of these different concepts, but as far as we are aware there has been no UK-wide or international work to define standards and definitions for care pathways. You might be forgiven for asking whether this matters. One could argue that provided the clinical team and local community that are developing and using the concept have their own localised working definition, then it doesn't matter. However, the lack of standards and definitions is, we feel, symptomatic of a lack of clarity of thinking and a systematic approach which impedes the speed of development and wastes time and effort on the part of the organisations trying to develop them. Such a lack of clarity typically leads to a wide variation in the type of care pathway developed and quality. As Cheah (1998)[32] points out, the resultant individual care pathway will be peculiar to the working culture, resources and knowledge of the organisation(s) that decide(s) to develop it and may contain biases in content as a result. This lack of clarity and definitions causes problems when specifying the functionality of computerised care pathway modules. Whilst you can work with a certain amount of ambiguity on paper-based care pathways because human beings are skilled at interpreting paper documents, in order to be able to translate pathways into a clinical computer system, there has to be rigour and consistency in the definition and use of the concepts which are applied to the design of the computer software.

Care pathways have spread from their initial introduction to healthcare in the US during the 1980s across many countries, including Australia, New Zealand, Japan and as well as several European countries. There is a difference of emphasis in the use of this concept by some of these different countries that is worth noting. For example, Currie and Harvey (2000),[1] Hainsworth *et al.* (1997),[33] Huber *et al.* (1998)[34] and Turley *et al.* (1994)[35] all point out that in the US, care pathways have been seen as a tool to control costs whilst maintaining the same level of quality and clinical outcomes. Sermeus *et al.* (2001)[36] argue that in Belgium and the Netherlands the emphasis is on cost containment and on developing patient-centred care. Latterly in Belgium they have concentrated on the achievement of clinical outcomes. Many of these care pathways take the form of check-lists of tasks and goals. In the UK the emphasis is on improving the quality of care, integrating services to make them reflect the patient's journey and acting as a model to ensure that best practice/clinical evidence (where available) and guidelines are implemented. In the UK the care pathway documentation often (although not always) replaces the individual patient clinical records and usually forms much more than simple check-lists. Despite these differences in emphasis we believe the concept described is essentially the same, it is just the local (national) context in which it is being implemented which varies.

Chapter 6 contains some proposals for national standards for care pathway and related concepts.

Conclusion

In this chapter we have argued that the current fragmentation of development and implementation of care pathways is hindering their take-up across the UK. We believe this situation is indicative of a fundamental problem with the limited way in which care pathways are perceived. Individuals tend to view the concept from their own particular domain, whereas we would argue that in order to have a significant impact on an organisation or the health service as a whole, we need to draw together the different perspectives of clinical, managerial and IT staff. Several limitations of care pathways (as they are being developed now) have been discussed. We believe that a systemic and systematic approach to draw together these different perspectives would provide significant advantages locally and from a national/international perspective.

The next chapter looks at the issue of knowledge management and keeping care pathways up to date with the latest clinical evidence.

References

1   Currie V and Harvey G (2000) The use of care pathways as tools to support the implementation of evidence-based practice. *Journal of Interprofessional Care.* **14**: 311–24.
2   Harkleroad A, Schirf D, Volpe J and Holm M (2000) Critical pathway development: an integrative literature review. *American Journal of Occupational Therapy.* **54**(2): 148–54.

3   Johnson S (1997) *Pathways of Care*. Blackwell Science, Oxford.

4   Ahgren B (2001) Chains of care: a counterbalance to fragmented healthcare. *Journal of Integrated Care Pathways*. **5**: 126–32.

5   Secretary of State for Health (2000) *The NHS Plan: a plan for investment, a plan for reform*. The Stationery Office, London.

6   Department of Health (2000) *National Service Framework for Coronary Heart Disease*. DoH, London.

7   Department of Health (2001) *National Service Framework for Older People*. DoH, London.

8   Pearson SD, Goulart-Fisher D and Lee TH (1995) Critical pathways as a strategy for improving care: problems and potential. *Annals of Internal Medicine*. **123**: 941–8.

9   Middleton S and Roberts A (2000) *Integrated Care Pathways: a practical approach to implementation*. Butterworth/Heinemann, Oxford.

10 de Luc K (2000) Care pathways – an evaluation of how effective they are. *Journal of Advanced Nursing*. **32**(2): 485–95.

11 Flower J, Geernaert M and Hartshorn A (2001) *Review of Issues and Options for Creating, Storing and Using Electronic Care Pathways across the NHS*. BBD Consultancy Services, Lichfield.

12 Morris AH (2000) Developing and implementing computerized protocols for standardization of clinical decisions. *Annals of Internal Medicine*. **132**: 373–83.

13 Grol R and Grimshaw JM (1999) Evidence-based implementation of evidence-based medicine. *Joint Community Journal of Quality Improvement*. **25**: 503–13.

14 Gross PA and Romano PS (2001) Introduction. *Medical Care*. **39**(8) Suppl 2: II-1.

15 NHS Centre For Reviews and Dissemination (1999) *Effective Health Care: getting evidence into practice* 5, 1. The Royal Society of Medicine Press Limited, London.

16 Campbell H, Hotchkiss R, Bradshaw N and Porteous M (1998) Integrated care pathways. *BMJ*. **316**: 133–7.

17 Layton A, Moss F and Morgan G (1998) Mapping out the patient's journey: experiences of developing pathways of care. *Quality in Health Care*. **7** (Suppl): S30–S36.

18 Togno-Armanasco V, Hopkin L and Harter S (1993) *Collaborative Nursing Case Management: a handbook for development and implementation*. Springer Publishing Company, New York.

19 March L, Cameron I, Cumming R, Chamberlain A, Schwarz J, Brnabic A *et al.* (2000) Mortality and morbidity after hip fracture: can evidence-based clinical pathways make a difference? *Journal of Rheumatology*. **27**(9): 2227–31.

20 de Luc K (2002) The ten-step guide to developing a care pathway. *Nurse 2 Nurse*. **2**(10): 10–12.

21 Clinical Systems Group (1998) *Improving Clinical Communications*. NHS Executive, Leeds.

22 Council of International Hospitals (1995) *Clinical Protocols: the clinical record*

Central Middlesex Hospital NHS Trust. The Advisory Board, Council of International Hospitals, London.

23 Lau C, Cartmill T and Leveaux V (1996) Managing and understanding variances in clinical path methodology: a case study. *Journal of Quality in Clinical Practice.* **16**: 109–17.

24 Hotchkiss R (1997) Integrated care pathways. *Nursing Times Research.* **2**: 30–6.

25 Currie L and Scrivener R (In press) Tracking care pathway activity across the UK National Health Service. *Journal of Clinical Excellence.*

26 Chu S (2001) Reconceptualising clinical pathway system design. *Collegian.* **8**(1): 33–6.

27 Dykes P (1998) *Psychiatric Clinical Pathways: an interdisciplinary approach.* Aspen Publishing, Maryland.

28 Jones T, de Luc K and Coyne H (1999) *Managing Care Pathways: the quality and resources of hospital care.* Association of Chartered Certified Accountants, London.

29 Every N, Hochman J, Becker R, Kopecky S and Cannon C (2000) Critical pathways: a review. *Circulation.* **101**: 461–5.

30 Trowbridge R and Weingarten S (2001) *Making Healthcare Safe: a critical analysis of patient safety practices.* Evidence Report/Technology Assessment, 2001, No. 43. Chapter 52. Prepared for the Agency for Healthcare Research and Quality. Website: www.ahcpr.gov/clinic/ptsafety/chap52.htm.

31 Johnson S (2001) What's in a name? *Journal of Integrated Care Pathways.* **5**(3): 111–12.

32 Cheah TS (1998) The impact of clinical guidelines and clinical pathways on medical practice: effectiveness and medico-legal aspects. *Annals of the Academy of Medicine.* **27**(4): 533–9.

33 Hainsworth D, Lockwood-Cook E, Pond M and Lagoe R (1997) Development and implementation of clinical pathways for stroke on a multi-hospital basis. *Journal of Neuroscience Nursing.* **29**(3): 156–62.

34 Huber T, Carlton L, Harward T, Russin M, Philips P, Nalli B *et al.* (1998). Impact of a clinical pathway for elective infrarenal aortic reconstructions. *Annals of Surgery.* **227**(5): 691–701.

35 Turley K, Tyndall M, Roge C, Cooper M, Turley K, Applebaum M *et al.* (1994) Critical pathway methodology: effectiveness in congenital heart surgery. *Annals of Thoracic Surgery.* **58**: 57–65.

36 Sermeus W, Vanhaecht K and Vleugels A (2001) The Belgian–Dutch clinical pathway network. *Journal of Integrated Care Pathways.* **5**: 10–14.

Part One

—

Knowledge management (clinical evidence)

Bertha Yuen Man Low and Pam Prior

Key points

- A methodology is outlined to assemble the knowledge base for the development and maintenance of a care pathway.

- There is a need to share the knowledge base for individual care pathways at a national level.

- A case study shows it is possible to link the knowledge base to a care pathway in an electronic format and to make it widely available.

Introduction

This chapter explores the contribution which knowledge management can make to the development of care pathways. It provides a methodology for assembling the knowledge base and in a case study shows how one can underpin a chest pain and myocardial infarction care pathway with the clinical evidence. It is argued that there is scope to make available this type of work at a national level so that individual healthcare organisations can gain from the efficiencies of sharing information.

'Knowledge, knowledge everywhere and nowhere left to think' (anon). This seems to be the reality created by the growth of clinical knowledge. The emphasis on the need to identify the evidence to underpin practice and critically appraising that evidence has added a new dimension to the demands of patient care and continuing professional development. It has also added a risk factor in the credibility of care pathways due to the difficulties in accessing up-to-date information. A recent study by Ely *et al.* (2002)[1] showed that individual clinicians still encounter up to 59 obstacles whilst searching for relevant information and using that information to direct patient care.

Care pathways are designed to support evidence-based practice but in order to do this they must be based on the latest evidence, always kept up to date and must make the evidence easily accessible to the clinical staff. The credibility of care pathways depends on the participants' acceptance of the choice of clinical evidence underpinning the treatment decisions. Whilst clinical experience will continue to guide these decisions, over the past decade some library and information professionals in the health sector have extended their traditional role and become knowledge members of the clinical team.

Role of the healthcare librarian

In addition to organising and giving structure to the knowledge anarchy, healthcare librarians mediate access to knowledge, interpreting and presenting information in a manner adjusted to the individual requirement of the clinician, ensuring all clinicians have equitable access to the knowledge base. This development has been supported by an increase in the production and use of resources to review and quality assess published evidence. These types of resources, in turn, are brought together under new knowledge 'portals' such as the National electronic Library for Health (www.nelh.nhs.uk) and the health education programme of subject-based portals, e.g. BIOME (www.biome.ac.uk).

NeLH is a prototype aiming to develop a digital library for NHS staff, patients and the public. NeLH includes signposting to significant, new evidence-based resources for health, e.g. the National Institute for Clinical Excellence (NICE) in addition to other less high-profile resources such as the Virtual Branch Libraries (VBLs).* These VBLs are created to foster electronic communities with a common interest, e.g. heart diseases. The Heart Diseases Virtual Branch Library** aims to bring together and index

---

* Renamed 'Specialist Libraries' from April 2003.
** Renamed 'Cardiovascular Diseases Specialist Library' from April 2003.

all the full text of documents from credible sources, published on the Internet. It also aims to find the best answers possible to real questions raised within clinical situations, by asking clinicians to put forward those questions and using all sources, electronic or otherwise, to create the best evidence-based answer possible from published information. VBLs are an experiment in encouraging open, multi-professional interaction in an electronic environment and are one component of a knowledge management environment with the potential to support the creation of care pathways.

Knowledge management is an evolving science. In the health sector much of the concentration of activity in this area is intended to give a framework to encourage the growth of IT skills in the workforce. When this has been achieved, the higher aims of knowledge management, which are to improve practice by sharing know-how, achieve rapid access to a core of accredited knowledge resources and encourage a community of practice to solve problems, will become realistic.

The clinicians, working with the clinical librarians or information professionals, will need to assemble the clinical knowledge base to inform the care pathway from its various components. The following five sections of this chapter explain the concepts and resources required to do this. These sections are: Identifying information needs; Information searching protocols; Searching for clinical guidelines; Critical appraisal of evidence and Updating the knowledge base.

Identifying information needs

According to de Luc (2002),[2] the detailed process for developing a care pathway involves ten steps and is outlined in full in Chapter 1 (Figure 1.1).

The ten steps to care pathway development include:

1 project plan the development
2 obtain information, including clinical evidence/guidelines
3 scope the care pathway
4 process map and redesign services
5 design the care pathway documentation
6 plan the changes in process
7 train the staff
8 test (or pilot) the care pathway
9 sign off the care pathway
10 ongoing maintenance/reviewing and updating of the care pathway.

There are few studies analysing the clinical information needs particularly related to the development of care pathways, but as a minimum steps two, three, four and five require access to the clinical evidence to inform the content of the care pathway.

As there has been little work identifying the clinical information needs for care pathway development, an alternative source of knowledge must be used to identify these requirements. As a substitute we can look to the evidence-based practice literature developed for clinical staff to provide some indication of the likely information needs. For example, Sackett et al. (2000)[3] identify ten categories of questions arising from clinical works, and Booth (2000)[4] classifies further the information needs of doctors by summarising various studies. These classifications can be used by the care pathway development team to provide a framework to search the clinical literature and check that they have included the information required within their individual care pathway templates (see Box 2.1).

Box 2.1 Information needs of clinicians

Sackett et al.[3]
Interpreting clinical
    findings
Aetiology
Presence of diseases or
    conditions
Differential diagnosis
Diagnostic tests
Prognosis
Therapy
Prevention
Experience and meaning
Self-improvement

Booth[4]
Therapy
• Dosage of drug
• Management of disease
• Treatment of disease
• Drug of choice
• Drug indications
• Identification of alternative therapies
• Improved quality of life for patient
    and/or family
• Confirmation of proposed therapy
• Minimisation of risks of treatment
• Revision of treatment plan
Diagnosis
• Presence of diseases or conditions
• Diagnostic tests
• Cause of test findings
• Recognition of abnormal or normal
    conditions
• Differential diagnosis
• Choice of diagnostic tests
Aetiology
Psychological effects
Audit of standards of care
Legal or ethical issues

Care pathways are task and goal-oriented plans for a specific clinical problem. The information needs identified indicate the critical steps along the process of care where support for decision making is needed. They will also bring out the gaps in knowledge for the development team, as well as the need for research.

When bringing the knowledge base together, the content must support the information needs of the care pathway, i.e.:

- about *the process of care* – there is a need to identify the information needs of clinicians along the process of care delivery
- about *supporting clinical decision making* – there is a need to investigate prescribed care, as well as alterations, and to incorporate multiple options (or branching) into care pathways
- about *putting evidence into practice* – there is a need to access, appraise and integrate various types of evidence into the care design, and to facilitate convenient links between care pathways and evidence
- about *providing information for the patient/carer* – there is a need to present information that is relevant and understandable
- about *providing information to support clinical audit and the monitoring of standards* – there is a need to collect information in a way that can be reviewed easily so that the care pathway can be updated as required.

Information searching protocols

In the context of planning care and knowledge management, Brown (2001)[5] argues care pathways represent point-of-care design which builds on pre-specified care. While pre-specified guidelines assure that planning care is evidence-based and effective, point-of-care design decides how and when to deliver the pre-specified guidelines and allows individualisation of care to achieve good patient outcomes.

In Figure 2.1, Brown outlines the various forms of evidence to be incorporated into pre-specification design and point-of-care design. This approach requires an information searching protocol to be set up to ensure all suitable sources of information are explored.

An information searching protocol is defined by Booth (2000)[4] as a tool defining 'the preferred route for particular types of enquiry determined by importance and likely yield of available sources'. The benefits of information searching protocols include:

- to make explicit the decision making in filtering evidence to support the care pathways

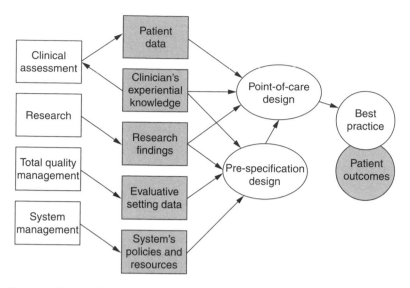

Figure 2.1 Brown's best practices healthcare map (2001).[5]

- to ensure comprehensive and systematic trawling of information sources for quality evidence, e.g. which databases to be used, which methodological filters to be applied etc.
- to document the search process
- to support future updating of the care pathways.

The design of information searching protocols requires the following components:

- knowledge of the patterns of potential information needs, e.g. what is the scope of the care pathways; what types of questions are raised by the development team
- knowledge of available sources and their strengths and weaknesses in coverage, e.g. which are the sources for established guidelines; what items are covered in a database and how they are selected.

The information searching protocols may adopt different foci and formats depending on the coverage of the care pathways. *Health Evidence Bulletins Wales*[6] includes a check-list of information sources and search strategies as part of the project methodology for compiling their recommendations. The School of Health and Related Research at the University of Sheffield (ScHARR)[7] has developed *Seeking the Evidence*, a suggested protocol for compiling evidence-based digests. Box 2.2 gives an example of a simplified searching protocol developed by the National electronic Library for Health, Heart Diseases Virtual

Box 2.2 Searching protocol for the Questions and Answers section of the Heart Diseases Virtual Branch Library pilot[8]

1 *Aims of the Q&As section*

The Q&As section aims to provide answers to common questions raised by healthcare workers. Where possible, links will be provided to existing reviews with some brief commentary summarising the main findings and possible application of the review. Where there is no existing review, a literature search will be undertaken and the main findings explained and summarised.

2 *Searching priorities*

Priority I

Systematic reviews, which synthesise evidence systematically, and official guidance with professional authority are sought first because they aim to provide comprehensive and unbiased advice.

Examples: Cochrane Database of Systematic Reviews; practice guidelines or scientific statements of professional organisations; health technology assessments etc.

Priority II

Other secondary research or sources appraising primary research that are relevant to the nature of the questions will be used next.

Examples: searching bibliographic databases, e.g. MEDLINE, EMBASE etc. for secondary research using methodological filters; sources appraising primary research include *Bandolier, ACP Journal Club* etc.

Priority III

If the above two criteria cannot be met, primary research will be used and appraised critically, and clinical trials will also be sought.

Examples: searching bibliographic databases, e.g. MEDLINE, EMBASE etc. for primary research using methodological filters; sources of clinical trials include National Research Registers etc.

3 *Other specifications*
- Methodological filters should be applied while searching for secondary and primary research from bibliographic databases.
- Full text of the evidence will be used in compiling the Q&As section.
- For health economics questions, refer to *Information Resources in Health Economics* (September 2000), compiled by the NHS Centre for Reviews and Dissemination/Centre for Health Economics of University of York, http://www.york.ac.uk/inst/crd/htadbase.htm.

Branch Library pilot site[8] for developing its Questions and Answers (Q&As) section.

Searching for clinical guidelines

Care pathways are proposed as a way of encouraging the translation of established clinical guidelines (or practice guidelines) into local practice. While care pathways include primary and secondary studies, and clinical expertise, as parts of the knowledge base, this section highlights particularly the application of clinical guidelines.

Clinical guidelines, like systematic reviews, are a type of secondary research which involves literature review, critical appraisal, multi-disciplinary consultation and grading of recommendations by level of evidence. Campbell *et al.* (1998)[9] made the point that clinical guidelines represent a form of strong evidence; however, their impact in improving healthcare is largely determined by local implementation.

Clinical guidelines are published by various organisations. In addition to printed literature, many are available on the Internet. The National Guideline Clearinghouse[10] and National electronic Library for Health Guideline Database[11] are initiatives facilitating repositories of clinical guidelines developed nationally, as well as locally. In addition there are tools developed to assess the quality of clinical guidelines, for example the AGREE[12] tool described by Cluzeau *et al.* (1999).[13] More sources for clinical guidelines are also available in Appendix 2.1.

For those published in printed literature only, conducting a literature search on bibliographic databases, e.g. MEDLINE, EMBASE, is required to identify them; and one can make use of methodological search filters to facilitate the trawling of clinical guidelines from databases.

Methodological search filters are validated search strategies using a combination of keywords and subject headings for retrieving literature of specific study designs and research methodologies. Various filters have been developed to achieve sensitivity or specificity in retrieval. Filters are usually database specific and should be added to subject searches, e.g. a search on 'asthma' combining with the filters for clinical guidelines. Box 2.3 gives an example of a methodological search filter for retrieving clinical guidelines developed by the London Library and Information Development Unit.[14]

Box 2.3 Methodological search filter for retrieving clinical guidelines from the MEDLINE database[14]

How to find guidelines and recommendations on MEDLINE using the Ovid search service:

1 guideline.pt
2 practice guideline.pt
3 (guideline$ or recommend$ or consensus).tw
4 (standards or parameter$).tw
5 exp guidelines
6 health planning/guidelines
7 1 or 2 or 3 or 4 or 5 or 6

Notes:

- Lines 1 and 2 search for publication types.
- Lines 3 and 4 search for words in the title or abstract.
- Line 5 searches for 'guidelines' or 'practice guidelines' as medical subject headings (MeSH).
- Line 6 searches for 'health planning guidelines' as medical subject headings (MeSH).

Critical appraisal of evidence

Sackett *et al.* (2000)[3] point out that the applicability of clinical guidelines to local communities depends on the extent to which they are in harmony or conflict with 'the killer Bs':

- *burden* of illness in terms of expected event rate.
- *beliefs* of the local communities about the value of the interventions.
- *bargain* in terms of cost of implementation.
- *barriers* in terms of geographic, organisational, traditional, authoritarian, legal or behavioural etc.

These factors are not only valid for clinical guidelines, but also true for the application of findings of primary and secondary research. To assist the assessment of the validity and usefulness of evidence, critical appraisal is called for to filter the evidence objectively and systematically.

Critical appraisal is also the stage where explicit knowledge in the form of published evidence and tacit knowledge (know-how) of clinicians' experience are combined for the development of care pathways. It decides whether the evidence is relevant to the specific stages of care or the

---

Box 2.4 Evaluating practice guidelines[15]

Are the results valid?

- Were all important options and outcomes specified?
- Was an explicit and sensible process used to identify, select and combine the evidence?
- Was an explicit and sensible process used to consider the relative value of different outcomes?
- Were important recent developments included?
- Has the guideline had peer review and testing?

What are the recommendations?

- Are practical, important recommendations made?
- How strong are the recommendations?
- Could the uncertainty in the evidence or values change the guideline's recommendations?

Will the results help me in patient care?

- Is the objective of the guideline consistent with mine?
- Are the recommendations applicable to my patients?

---

specific needs of clinicians at the specific point of delivering care, whether there is a need to take into consideration expert opinions or local needs, or whether there are gaps in research.

Various appraisal check-lists have been developed for different types of clinical questions and study designs. Box 2.4 provides an example of the critical appraisal check-list for clinical guidelines from the University of Alberta.[15]

Updating the knowledge base

Campbell *et al.* (1998)[9] point out that any development programme of care pathways should have a robust mechanism to collect and analyse variances, update the pathways by incorporating agreed changes and identify research issues. Apart from including the evidence in the documentation of the care pathways, updating the knowledge base should form part of the regular review.

Current awareness services provide information users with the latest news within their chosen subject areas or interests and are available via various sources, some of which are fee based and some freely available. A sample of such services includes:

- specific current awareness service providers, e.g. ZETOC developed by the British Library[16] – these service providers have their own bibliographic databases; users may specify their interests by broad subject categories, keywords, journal titles or simple search strategies
- search alert function supported by individual search services, e.g. Ovid,[17] PubMed[18] – such function is based on the search strategies saved on individual bibliographic databases; users may specify their interests by a variety of search methods, including complicated search strategies
- current awareness services available on websites of individual journals, or information aggregators, or organisations, e.g. BMJ,[19] CatchWord[20] – these services usually provide updates on new additions to their websites only
- personalisation supported by individual websites, e.g. BBC[21] – certain websites allow users to customise the types of information to be displayed; the information on pre-selected subject categories is updated each time you visit the websites.

The appendices at the end of this chapter show two diagrams and their associated website listings. Appendix 2.1, called '12 reasons for surfing the Internet' lists different types of information resource available on the web. Appendix 2.2, called 'Tools for resource discovery', lists tools available on the web that will help you find other information resources. Many of the sites in the second diagram provide collections of Internet addresses. These diagrams focus on obtaining primarily clinical information. Please note information resources relating to the actual development process of care pathways covering aspects of change management, facilitation etc. are provided in Chapter 3. Also, at the end of this book is a list of general websites relating specifically to care pathways.

Assembling the knowledge base to underpin the development of care pathways is complex and time-consuming and requires expertise. Rather than each organisation or health community starting this process from the beginning, it would seem more efficient to do something on a national level that can be made available to all healthcare organisations. They could then review and localise the information as required. The next section of this chapter explores a basic example of this, where the knowledge management underpinning a particular care pathway was made available electronically on the web using the Heart Diseases Virtual Branch Library.

A case study: linking a chest pain and myocardial infarction care pathway with the knowledge base

The Partnership for Developing Quality[22] and the National electronic Library for Health Heart Diseases Virtual Branch Library pilot site[8] have been working together to develop a model to link care pathways with their supporting knowledge base electronically. The project aimed to support the local adaptation of the generic 'chest pain and myocardial infarction pathway' developed for the West Midlands health community, and to encourage an evidence-based approach in developing and implementing care pathways.

The 'chest pain and myocardial infarction pathway' will be made available electronically on the Heart Diseases Virtual Branch Library website. Note that this example shows early steps in a relatively basic software environment.

In order to link the care pathway with the knowledge base, the stages of care outlined in the care pathway paper documentation (which is used to record actual patient care) are summarised diagrammatically in the form of a process map. This process map identifies the sequence of planned interventions and main decision points. An example of the translation between the care pathway documentation and the process map is shown in Figure 2.2.

The next stage is to link the process map which underpins the care pathway document to the supporting knowledge base. This is illustrated in Figure 2.3. By using simple hyperlinks, each stage of the pathway process map is linked to a summary of appraised evidence and any related information for the patient. The original documents of both the evidence and the patient information can also be displayed by simply activating the embedded hyperlinks on the VBL.

The project is still at an early stage offering limited functionality; however, it demonstrates an approach to incorporating the knowledge base in the development and presentation as well as the application of care pathways.

Effectively the presentation of clinical knowledge is available in four layers:

- the care pathway documentation
- the process map
- the summary of evidence
- the full detail of the evidence and accredited patient information.

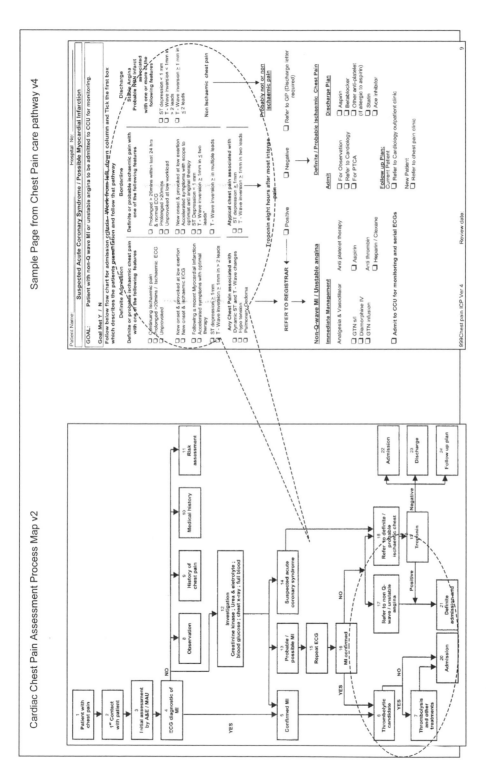

Figure 2.2 Example of relationship between process map and care pathway documentation.

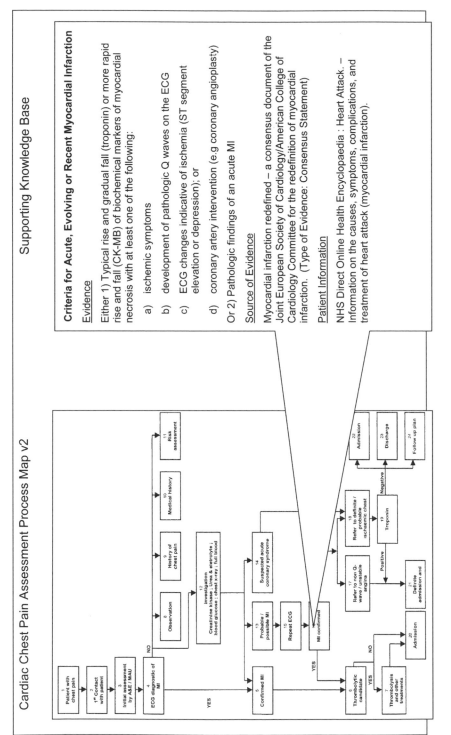

Figure 2.3 The model of the Heart Diseases Virtual Branch Library in linking care pathways and the knowledge base.

Providing the layers allows for day-to-day discussions, and more detailed information to follow up research or to supplement training or continuing professional development.

An advantage of using the VBL as the basis of the work is that it is a reliable, regularly updated, quality-checked resource, with its hyperlinks tested to ensure no dislocations occur. There is the need for common policies between the VBL and the care pathway in electronic form to ensure any changes to one are picked up by the other. This could be something as simple as a broken hyperlink, which is easily avoided by regular use of hyperlink checking software. It could also be the presentation of updated evidence, which might change the decisions within the pathway.

Although not active at this point of development, the next step might be an additional action to add to the summary to initiate a predetermined search strategy on the VBL database, alerting to records with matching concepts. This will ensure that any new evidence is presented as it becomes available.

In summary, to enable this to happen (*see* Glossary for explanation of technical terms):

- the Heart Diseases Virtual Branch Library is database driven, using Active Server Pages to present the web pages
- the records in the database have keywords based on MeSH
- the patient information is available as flat HTML from EQUIP,[23] a patient information site
- the summary information is created manually using HTML then hyperlinked to the care pathway process map, which has been set up as an image map. This is then hyperlinked to other more detailed resources using the VBL as the knowledge base.

Changing access arrangements to health knowledge in the UK

In an ideal electronic world, gaining access to published knowledge should be easier than ever before. In reality there is a long way to go, partly because some scholarly publications see a loss of revenue in converting to electronic access. The market has added layers of complexity in what can, or cannot, be made readily available in what format. Unlike higher education, the NHS is not mature in electronic knowledge resource procurement. As a result, different parts of the health service in the UK provide different resources and users often have a whole portfolio of usernames and passwords to use to gain access to subscription-based resources.

At this time (late 2002) there is an initiative to achieve centralised procurement of resources, linked through a National Knowledge Service.[24] This should help to stabilise electronic access and build new relationships with publishers. There is also a trend towards the use of the Athens Authentication Service,[25] with the opportunity to simplify usernames and passwords.

Copyright is an additional complexity. All published information, whether in paper or electronic formats, is copyrighted and will have restrictions on its use. The NHS in England has an agreement with the Copyright Licensing Agency,[26] which allows some multiple copying of paper resources. Before making hyperlinks to journal articles or books in electronic form, the conditions of the licence and the current negotiations on copyright must be checked and arrangements for any additional permissions put in place.

A promising development towards direct electronic access to evidence comes in the form of the Digital Object Identifier (DOI) standard.[27] This is a global electronic indexing system, similar in principle to the way in which web servers are found by their 'domain name' (e.g. nelh.nhs.uk), or the ISBN system for cataloguing books. Each file in the DOI system is assigned a unique reference number. When this number is submitted to an independent Internet service, it sends back the location of the document. If the DOI reference number for a particular document was embedded in a computerised care pathway, the evidence could be displayed on demand within seconds, which would be a significant aid to decision support.

Conclusion

Providing a seamless knowledge management environment to underpin a care pathway requires a mix of different skills. Some elements may be managed through a web-based interface and this will increase, of necessity, as more resources become available in this medium. This chapter shows the potential for escalating the pace of change, through partnership working involving clinicians, NeLH, information professionals responsible for national procurement and specialist services and locally based clinical librarians.

In the Introduction to this book the problem of unnecessary replication of effort at the local organisational or clinical team level was discussed. Care pathways that cover the same conditions/disease groups should have a similar evidence base. There is an urgent need to co-ordinate the searching for this evidence base on a national level and for the results to be made accessible to all healthcare organisations.

References

1   Ely J, Osheroff J and Ebell M (2002) Obstacles to answering doctors' questions about patient care with evidence: qualitative study. *BMJ*. **324**: 710–24.
2   de Luc K (2002) The ten-step guide to developing a care pathway. *Nurse 2 Nurse*. **2**(10): 10–12.
3   Sackett DL, Straus SE, Richardson WS, Rosenberg W and Haynes RB (2000) Asking answerable clinical questions. In: DL Sackett *et al.* (eds) *Evidence-based Medicine: how to practise and teach EBM* (2e). Churchill Livingstone, Edinburgh.
4   Booth A (2000) Selecting appropriate sources. In: A Booth and G Walton (eds) *Managing Knowledge in Health Services*. Library Association Publishing, London.
5   Brown SJ (2001) Managing the complexity of best practice healthcare. *Journal of Nursing Care Quality*. **15**(2): 1–8.
6   Health Evidence Bulletins Wales *Project Methodology 4*. http://hebw.uwcm. ac.uk/projectmethod/index.htm.
7   University of Sheffield School of Health and Related Research (ScHARR) *Seeking the Evidence: a protocol*. http://www.shef.ac.uk/~scharr/ir/proto.html.
8   National electronic Library for Health Heart Diseases Virtual Branch Library pilot site, http://www.wish-uk.org/znelh.
9   Campbell H, Hotchkiss R, Bradshaw N and Porteous M (1998) Care pathways. *BMJ*. **316**: 133–7.
10 National Guideline Clearinghouse, http://www.guideline.gov.
11 National electronic Library for Health Guideline Database, http://www.nelh.nhs.uk.
12 AGREE Guideline Appraisal Instrument (2001), http://www.agreecollaboration. org/appraisal.html.
13 Cluzeau F, Littlejohns P, Grimshaw J, Feder G and Moran S (1999) Development and application of a generic methodology to assess the quality of clinical guidelines. *International Journal for Quality in Health Care*. **11**: 21–8.
14 London Library and Information Development Unit (LIDU) *Methodological Filters for Retrieving Guidelines and Recommendations on MEDLINE*. http://www.londonlinks.ac.uk/evidence_strategies/ovid_filters.htm.
15 University of Alberta *Evidence-based Medicine Toolkit*. http://www.med. ualberta.ca/ebm/ebm.htm.
16 ZETOC: electronic table of contents from the British Library, http://zetoc. mimas.ac.uk/.
17 Ovid, http://www.ovid.com.
18 PubMed, http://www.ncbi.nih.gov/entrez/query.fcgi.
19 BMJ, http://bmj.com/.
20 CatchWord, http://www.catchword.co.uk/journalalert.htm.
21 BBC, http://www.bbc.co.uk/.
22 Partnership for Developing Quality, http://www.wmpdq.org/index.html.

23 Electronic Information for Patients, http://equip.nhs.uk/.

24 National Knowledge Service, http://www.doh.gov.uk/ipu/whatnew/itevent/tables/nationalknowledgeservice.htm.

25 Athens Authentication Service, http://www.athens.ac.uk.

26 Copyright Licensing Agency, http://www.cla.co.uk.

27 The Digital Object Identifier System, International DOI Foundation, http://www.doi.org.

Appendix 2.1: Twelve reasons for surfing the Internet

This appendix lists some useful Internet resources in 12 categories:

1 Review of primary research
2 Digest of primary research
3 Guidelines and guideline appraisal tools
4 Clinical trials
5 Drug information
6 Primary research
7 Participating in virtual communities
8 Official information
9 Education and training
10 Patient information
11 News
12 Web evaluation.

Figure 2A1.1 provides an overview of these resources.

1 Review of primary research

- Cochrane Library (NeLH), http://www.nelh.nhs.uk
- DARE (Database of Abstracts of Reviews of Effectiveness), http://agatha.york.ac.uk/darehp.htm
- HTA (NHS R&D Health Technology Assessment Programme), http://www.hta.nhsweb.nhs.uk/htapubs.htm
- NHSEED (NHS Economic Evaluation Database), http://agatha.york.ac.uk/nhsdhp.htm
- NHSCRD (NHS Centre for Reviews and Dissemination) systematic reviews, http://www.york.ac.uk/inst/crd/srinfo.htm
- Effectiveness Health Care bulletins, http://www.york.ac.uk/inst/crd/ehcb.htm
- Effectiveness Matters, http://www.york.ac.uk/inst/crd/em.htm

2 Digest of primary research

- Bandolier, http://www.jr2.ox.ac.uk/bandolier/index.html
- ACP Journal Club, http://www.acpjc.org/
- CAT Banks, http://www.minervation.com/cebm/docs/catbank.html
- EBM (Evidence-based Medicine), http://ebm.bmjjournals.com/

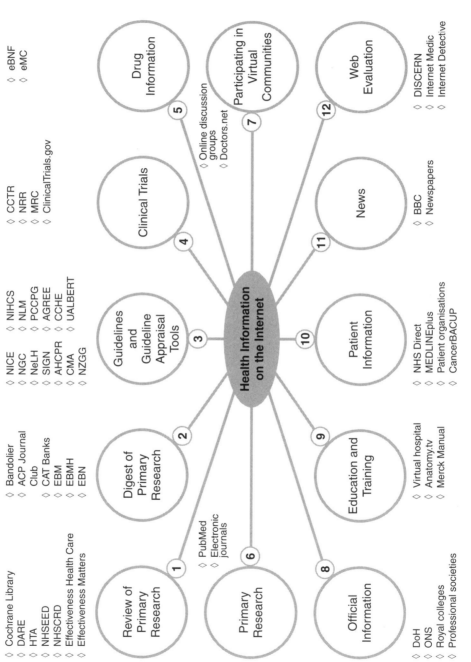

Figure 2A1.1 Twelve reasons for surfing the Internet.

- EBMH (Evidence-based Mental Health), http://www.acponline.org/journals/ebm/
- EBN (Evidence-based Nursing), http://ebn.bmjjournals.com/

3 Guidelines

- NICE (National Institute for Clinical Excellence), http://www.nice.org.uk/
- NGC (National Guideline Clearinghouse), http://www.guidelines.gov/
- NeLH (National electronic Library for Health), http://www.nelh.nhs.uk/
- SIGN (Scottish Intercollegiate Guidelines Network), http://www.sign.ac.uk/guidelines/index.html
- Agency for Health Care Research and Quality, http://www.ahcpr.gov/
- Canadian Medical Association Clinical Practice Guidelines Database, http://www.cma.ca/
- National electronic Library for Health MPG eguidelines, http://www.nelh.nhs.uk/
- New Zealand Guidelines Group, http://www.nzgg.org.nz/library.cfm
- National Institute of Health Consensus Statements, http://odp.od.nih.gov/consensus/
- NLM health services/technology assessment text, http://text.nlm.nih.gov/
- Primary care clinical practice guidelines, http://medicine.ucsf.edu/resources/guidelines/index.html

Guideline appraisal tools

- AGREE: appraising the quality of clinical guidelines, http://www.sign.ac.uk/methodology/agreeguide/
  The AGREE pro forma or check-list helps make an informed judgement about the methods that were used to develop a guideline.
- Centre for Health Evidence: users' guides to evidence-based practice, http://www.cche.net/usersguides/main.asp
  Offers the complete collection of *Users' Guides to Evidence-based Practice*, originally published as a series in the *Journal of the American Medical Association (JAMA)*.
- University of Alberta: evidence-based medicine toolkit, http://www.med.ualberta.ca/ebm/ebm.htm
  Offers evaluation tools, search guides and worksheets for different types of clinical questions.

4 Clinical trials

- CCTR (Cochrane Controlled Trials Register) (NeLH), http://www.nelh.nhs.uk/
- NRR (National Research Register), http://www.update-software.com/National/
- MRC (Medical Research Council), http://fundedresearch.cos.com/MRC/
- ClinicalTrials.gov, http://clinicaltrials.gov/

5 Drug information

- eBNF (Electronic British National Formulary), http://www.bnf.org/
- eMC (Electronic Medical Compendium), http://emc.vhn.net/

6 Primary research

- PubMed, http://www.ncbi.nlm.nih.gov/entrez/query.fcgi
- Electronic journals:
  - FreeMedicalJournals.com, http://www.freemedicaljournals.com/
  - Directory of Electronic Health Services Journals, http://www.freemedicaljournals.com/
  - websites of libraries

7 Participating in virtual communities

- Online discussion groups:
  - National Academic Mailing List Service, http://www.freemedicaljournals.com/
  - Smartgroups, http://www.smartgroups.com/care-pathways
  - Informatics Learning Networks, http://www.ecommunity.nhs.uk
- Doctors.net, http://www.doctors.net/

8 Official information

- DoH (Department of Health), http://www.doh.gov.uk/
- ONS (Office of National Statistics), http://www.statistics.gov.uk/
- Royal Colleges:
  - Royal College of General Practitioners, http://www.rcgp.org.uk/
  - Royal College of Nursing, http://www.rcgp.org.uk/
  - Royal College of Obstetricians and Gynaecologists, http://www.rcog.org.uk/

- Royal College of Physicians of Edinburgh, http://www.rcpe.ac.uk/library/index.html
- Royal College of Physicians of London, http://www.rcplondon.ac.uk/college/library/index.htm
- Royal College of Psychiatrists, http://www.rcpsych.ac.uk/info/index.htm
- Royal College of Surgeons of Edinburgh, http://www.rcsed.ac.uk/geninfo/library/Default.asp
- Royal College of Surgeons of England, http://www.rcseng.ac.uk/services/library/
- Royal Society of Medicine, http://www.roysocmed.ac.uk/librar/library.htm
- Professional societies

9 Education and training

- Virtual hospital, http://www.vh.org/
- Anatomy.tv (NeLH), http://www.nelh.nhs.uk/
- Merck Manual, http://www.merck.com/pubs/mmanual/

10 Patient information

- NHS Direct online, http://www.nhsdirect.nhs.uk/
- MEDLINEplus, http://www.medlineplus.gov/
- CancerBACUP, http://www.cancerbacup.org.uk
- MIDIRS/NeLH Informed Choice, http://www.nelh. nhs.uk
  (Follow the MIDIRS link on the left-hand frame and click on leaflets – this will provide useful obstetric information for patients.)

11 News

- BBC, http://www.bbc.co.uk/
- Newspapers:
  - directory of UK newspapers, http://www.bubl.ac.uk/uk/newspapers.htm

12 Web evaluation

- DISCERN: quality criteria for consumer health information, http://www.discern.org.uk/
- Internet Medic, http://omni.ac.uk/vts/medic/
- Internet Detective, http://www.sosig.ac.uk/desire/internet-detective.html

Appendix 2.2: Tools for resource discovery

This appendix lists tools available on the web which will help you find other information resources. Many of these sites provide collections of Internet addresses.

These sites are in seven categories:

1 Bibliographic databases
2 Library websites
3 Subject gateways: patient information
4 Subject gateways: medical information
5 Subject gateways: nursing and allied health information
6 Internet search engines
7 Specialist search tools and methodological search filters.

Figure 2A2.1 provides an overview of these resources.

1 Bibliographic databases

- PubMed, http://www.ncbi.nlm.nih.gov/entrez/query.fcgi
- MEDLINE, http://www.nlm.nih.gov/databases/databases_medline. html
  Content also accessible via PubMed; enquire at local libraries.
- EMBASE (Excepta Medica Database), http://www.elsevier.com/ locate/embase
  Access at cost; enquire at local libraries.
- CINAHL (Cumulative Index to Nursing and Allied Health Literature), http://www.cinahl.com/
  Access at cost; enquire at local libraries.
- PsychLIT (Psychiatry and Psychology Database), http://www.psycinfo. com/
  Access at cost; enquire at local libraries.
- CancerLit, http://www.nci.nih.gov/search/cancer_literature/
- AMED (Allied and Complementary Health Database), http:// www.bl.uk/services/information/amed.html
  Access at cost; enquire at local libraries.
- Caredata: the social care knowledge base, http://www.elsc.org.uk/ bases_floor/caredata.htm
- PEDro (Physiotherapy Evidence Database), http://ptwww.cchs.usyd. edu.au/pedro/

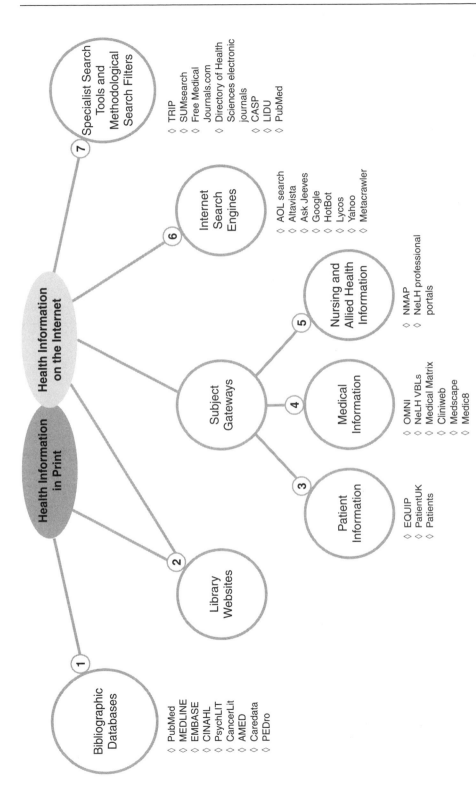

Figure 2A2.1 Tools for resource discovery.

2 Library websites

Provide collections of Internet addresses.

3 Subject gateways: patient information

- EQUIP (Electronic Quality Information for Patients), http://www.equip.nhs.uk/
- Patient UK, http://www.patient.co.uk
- Patients, http://www.patients.org.uk

4 Subject gateways: medical information

- OMNI, http://omni.ac.uk/
- NeLH VBLs (National electronic Library for Health Virtual Branch Libraries),* http://www.nelh.nhs.uk/
- Cliniweb, http://www.cliniweb.com/
- Medical Matrix, http://www.medmatrix.org/
- Medscape, http://www.medscape.com/
- Medic8, http://www.medic8.com

5 Subject gateways: nursing and allied health information

- NMAP, http://nmap.ac.uk/
- NeLH professional portals, http://www.nelh.nhs.uk/

6 Internet search engines

- AOL search, http://search.aol.com
- Altavista, http://www.altavista.com
- Ask Jeeves, http://www.askjeeves.com
- Google, http://www.google.com
- HotBot, http://www.hotbot.com
- Lycos, http://www.lycos.com
- Yahoo, http://www.yahoo.com
- Metacrawler, http://www.metacrawler.com

---

* Renamed 'Specialist Libraries' from April 2003.

7 *Specialist search tools*

- TRIP (Turning Research into Practice database), http://www. tripdatabase.com/
- SUMsearch, http://sumsearch.uthscsa.edu/searchform45.htm
- Free Medical Journals.com, http://www.freemedicaljournals.com/
- Directory of Health Sciences electronic journals, http://www.hunter. health.nsw.gov.au/index.php?p=100

Methodological search filters

- CASPfew: filters, http://wwwlib.jr2.ox.ac.uk/caspfew/filters/filters.html Offers methodological search filters for searching MEDLINE, CINAHL, EMBASE, PSYCHINFO.
- LIDU (London Library and Information Development Unit): methodological filters, http://www.londonlinks.ac.uk/evidence_strategies/index.htm Offers methodological search filters for searching MEDLINE.
- PubMed: clinical queries using research methodology filters, http://www.ncbi.nlm.nih.gov/entrez/query/static/clinical.html Offers methodological search filters for searching MEDLINE on PubMed.

3

Care pathway development

Chris Homer and Linda Dunn

Key points

- Development of 'generic' care pathways is possible as long as ownership of the care pathway is achieved locally.

- Key considerations when managing change as part of a care pathway development are:
  - how to influence people
  - how to deal with resistance
  - how to negotiate and build consensus
  - leadership
  - facilitation.

- A multifaceted approach to implementation is required to change behaviour. Care pathways utilise a range of implementation techniques.

Introduction

Gaining consensus on care pathway content is fraught with difficulties. Ensuring that the care pathway is successfully developed and implemented requires an understanding of the organisational, professional, personal and interpersonal barriers to change and how to overcome them.

This chapter discusses the management of change in the NHS and the skills and competencies required by individuals and teams involved in the development and implementation of care pathways. By way of illustration, three different approaches to care pathway development are described and reference is made to sources of assistance, learning and support.

Care pathways in the context of the change agenda

Plamping (1998)[1] said that despite almost continual reform since its inception in 1948, many see the NHS as unchanging. Reforms generally deal with structural and organisational change when, in reality, changing the NHS involves changing the behaviour of individuals and groups. To argue that clinical practice has not changed since 1948 is clearly difficult, but because this change focuses around individual clinicians and small teams it is incremental, occurs in isolation and spreads slowly. Despite large amounts of literature supporting evidence-based healthcare, ineffective practices continue and effective practices are not always used. This phenomenon precedes the NHS; Haines and Jones (1994)[2] cite Lancaster's evidence of 1601 for the effectiveness of lemon juice in the prevention of scurvy and the eventual adoption of its use by the Navy in 1795. This phenomenon continues in more recent times, as pointed out by Antman *et al.* (1992),[3] with the long delay between the consistent publication and application of the benefits of thrombolitic treatment in myocardial infarction.

The policy-driven change of today strives to improve the quality, efficiency and accountability of healthcare and requires widespread transformational change involving whole systems of healthcare delivery.

Gordon (1995)[4] makes the point that care pathways are a tool that can help to change clinical practice. They determine the clinical component of a healthcare process, promote the implementation of evidence-based healthcare and improve performance rather than just process. They assist multi-professional groups to analyse and evaluate the interactions between uni-professional inputs and therefore begin to address the clinical aspects of the multiple processes of healthcare, making a step towards transformational change and involving organisational restructuring, process simplification and redesign, and systems redesign. This is shown diagrammatically in Figure 3.1.

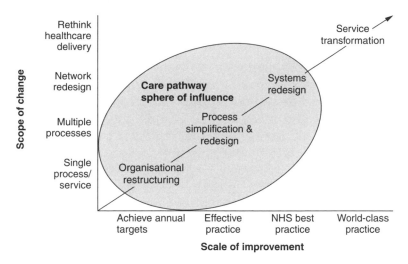

Figure 3.1 Position of care pathways in the progression to transformational change.

Care pathway development and a regional case study

This case study provides a summary of one region's experiences with trying different approaches to the development of care pathways. A more detailed analysis is provided in Appendix 3.1. This work was supported and funded by the Partnership for Developing Quality, West Midlands, which existed to promote and share best practice across the region. The case study involves the testing of three distinct approaches to care pathway development undertaken over a two-year period from 2000 to 2002.

The Partnership for Developing Quality facilitated the development of care pathways in three areas across the region, namely, learning disabilities, coronary heart disease and stroke services. Its aim was to avoid reinventing the wheel by all the individual healthcare trusts and primary care trusts (PCTs) who were doing work separately and to share and promote good practice across the region. In summary, the three different projects were:

1 **Learning disabilities** – four care pathways were developed in challenging behaviour, epilepsy, hearing impairment and transitions from child to adult services. You can read more about the detail of these individual care pathways in the following articles: Ahmad et al. (2002),[5] Brady et al. (2002),[6] Pitts et al. (2002)[7] and Ahmad et al. (2002).[8]

The approach taken for the development of these care pathways was as follows:

- A multi-professional steering group was established.
- A project manager and four individual care pathway facilitators were identified who had dedicated time for this project.
- Multidisciplinary and multi-agency groups with representatives from across the region and user groups met regularly to develop the regional 'generic' care pathways in the four topic areas. (For the purposes of this project a 'generic' pathway meant one developed for a particular group of clients, e.g. those suffering from epilepsy, which could be implemented in multiple healthcare organisations across the region.)
- The care pathways were tested (unchanged) in pilot sites around the region.
- The work was the first of its kind in the region – very little work had been undertaken in care pathways in this speciality before and in identifying the evidence base for many of the common practices performed in these areas.

2 **Coronary heart disease** – the care pathway for chest pain and myocardial infarction. The approach taken for the development of this care pathway was as follows:

- A multi-professional project steering group with user representation was established.
- A dedicated facilitator was identified to project manage the development.
- A multidisciplinary group with representatives from across the region met regularly to develop a regional 'generic' care pathway with the aim of it being implemented in multiple healthcare organisations across the region.
- The 'generic' care pathway was localised and tested in pilot sites around the region.
- A wide range of work had already been undertaken by various organisations throughout the region on this topic. Some organisations had developed process maps whilst others had already developed and were using their own locally developed pathways. The challenge was to see if these organisations would participate in the development of a 'generic' pathway underpinned by the National Service Framework for Coronary Heart Disease (2000)[9] and share their knowledge on local practice.

3 **Stroke services** – the care pathway covered prevention, immediate care, early and continuing rehabilitation, and long-term support for all those

suffering from stroke. The approach taken for the development of the care pathway was as follows:

- A project management group, including a number of stroke co-ordinators and care pathway facilitators from around the region, was established.
- There was no dedicated facilitator.
- The group wanted a mechanism that would facilitate the process of shared learning between organisations across the region and that would help them develop their *own* local care pathway for each participating organisation. The aim was not to produce a generic pathway but rather that links should be made between primary/secondary/tertiary care across all professional and appropriate agencies around the region.
- An electronic network was established to facilitate the sharing of information on an ongoing basis. This meant it was only necessary to have a limited number of workshop meetings at three to four-monthly intervals.
- Organisations were at varying stages in their development of a stroke care pathway. A small number had a pathway running locally, a few had started development and most planned to start development shortly.
- The organisations participating wanted to develop a stroke pathway in each of their respective organisations which was underpinned by the *National Service Framework for Older People* (2001).[10]

Lessons learnt from comparing these three approaches

- The approach adopted for development must suit the stage that the contributing organisations are at with their own development of a care pathway.
- The less work done in the area previously by organisations on an individual basis, the easier it is to adopt a regional approach and develop a 'generic' pathway which can be used across multiple sites.
- It is possible to develop generic pathways whilst achieving local ownership, but much depends on the attitude of the multi-professional group to this approach.
- It is not always possible to obtain agreement on which clinical evidence should inform the content of the care pathway (in spite of national guidelines and evidence-based practice).
- Dedicated facilitation time to progress the development is essential. Even if electronic networking alternatives are used, these require considerable effort to set up and implement effectively. Electronic

networks do not necessarily speed up the process of pathway development and implementation of change.

The case study reflects many of the human issues surrounding a change management project. The rest of this chapter discusses these important issues. It identifies how care pathways can act as a change management tool and also what is required to increase the likelihood of achieving the successful development and implementation of them.

Managing change

Much has been written on the theory of change and change management and it is not the place of this chapter to repeat it all again. However, the large volume of literature makes it difficult for clinicians and managers involved in the implementation of change to assess where their focus should be. The National Coordinating Centre for NHS Service Delivery and Organisation (NCCSDO) (2001)[11], (2001)[12] has reviewed existing research findings of relevance to change management and quality improvement in the NHS and published two comprehensive resource and reference tools. These are available on the web in downloadable form from www.sdo.lshtm.ac.uk. They are recommended as sources of tools and information to aid the implementation of change and allow this chapter to focus its attention on interpersonal rather than theoretical aspects of change.

Achieving and sustaining change will require new skills and competencies throughout the NHS. Newman *et al.* (1998)[13] adopted the premise that it is even more difficult to change the behaviour of others than of yourself, and defined key competencies for those leading a change in clinical practice that included:

- personal attributes
  - leadership
  - adaptability
  - commitment to secure change
- interpersonal skills
  - communication
  - negotiation
  - influencing
  - multi-professional working
- self-management skills
  - time management
- information management
  - technical knowledge and skills.

Influencing people

One of the main barriers to the implementation of care pathways is where changes in clinical behaviour are required.

Oppenheim (1992)[14] said, 'We can not necessarily predict behaviour from attitudes; nor are attitudes readily inferred from behaviour with any validity . . .'

People's behaviour is related to their values, attitudes and beliefs, but not necessarily dependent on them. The behaviours and modes of thinking which determine the way an individual reacts to their environment characterise an individual's personality. Clearly, influencing behaviour is a complex task but will be made easier by an awareness of environmental factors and how they impact on those we are trying to influence, an understanding of the behavioural patterns of those involved including ourselves and an analysis of how these factors might conflict and complement.

A considerable amount of study has explored the relationship between behaviours and personality characteristics. Five major approaches to personality have emerged. These are:

- psychoanalytic
- type
- trait
- social learning
- humanistic.

All the approaches seek to develop a model of the person that will, systematically, account for their unique underlying personality structure and in so doing provide a framework allowing us to understand individuals and compare them with each other. Carl Jung (1971),[15] who was primarily from the psychoanalytic school, was the first to classify people into psychological types and made the distinction between introversion and extroversion. Isabel Myers and Katherine Briggs extended Jung's classifications to develop the Myers–Briggs Type Indicator (1987),[16] a frequently used questionnaire which determines 16 types of personality from four basic preferences. It is not practical to apply this sort of tool to determine the personality type of all stakeholders involved in the care pathway development. However, an awareness of these personality types helps us identify how we might influence individuals in the change process. Further sources of information on the Myers–Briggs tool are provided in the final section of this chapter.

From observation of those around us, four broad behavioural styles can be identified: the analyst, the driver, the amiable and the enthusiast. None of these styles is 'better' than any of the others and in reality, although we all have a preferred style, it is possible to change styles and exert a different influence on those around us. When played to their strengths the different styles complement each other and enhance the work of a team. Too often there is a focus on the 'differences' between individual viewpoints and an intolerance of their preferred way of working which results in conflict and diminishes the output of the team.

Teamworking

West and Field (1995)[17] point out that '. . . nearly a century of research on team working within organisational psychology suggests that there are real difficulties in achieving effective teamwork'.

Research has repeatedly highlighted the failure of teams to perform better than the aggregate of the individual members. West and Slater (1995)[18] attribute this to the tendency of some members to exert less effort in a team than they would as an individual whilst still believing that the efforts of others will be enough to achieve the task. Others, perceiving the inequity of effort, may reduce their effort so as not to become the victims of the 'free wheelers'. When individuals focus on themselves rather than the team, teamwork is not effective. Guzzo and Shea (1992)[19] argue teams are most effective when:

- individuals feel that they are important to the fate of the group
- individual tasks are meaningful and intrinsically rewarding
- individual contributions are identifiable and subject to evaluation and comparison
- teams have intrinsically interesting tasks to perform
- there are clear group goals and built-in performance feedback.

The successful development and implementation of care pathways involves engaging with stakeholders from multi-professional groups, clarifying the rationale for actions taken and gaining consensus on evidence and best practice. Firth-Cousins (1998)[20] argues that as an exercise in itself this should improve working across the wider team. West (1994)[21] describes the determinants of the quality of innovation in teamwork as:

- clarity of team objectives
- level of participation (information sharing, interaction and influence over decision making)
- task orientation (constructive controversy, commitment to excellence)
- practical support for innovation.

To be successful in developing a care pathway the team must try to develop these features.

It is interesting to note that a similar set of requirements is outlined later in this book in Chapter 5 (*see* p. 118) by Mayer when examining the reasons for business process re-engineering failures. This illustrates how the systems literature reports similar conclusions to the change management literature, but from a different perspective.

Implementation strategies

There is a growing body of research evidence about the effectiveness of strategies to implement research findings into practice. Many approaches to implementation have been suggested. Haines and Jones (1994)[2] whilst expressing the opinion that 'the implementation of research findings can not be left solely to spontaneous local initiatives' also felt that 'a top-down, centralised approach to implementation is unlikely to achieve changes in behaviour'. They acknowledged a place for both approaches and proposed a wide-reaching system of integration. Batstone and Edwards (1996)[22] considered that project management assisted the implementation of evidence by linking guideline development to the business cycle, whereas Dunning *et al.* (1998)[23] advocated a move from a project-based to a systems-based approach in order to secure and sustain changes in clinical practice.

Grimshaw *et al.* (2001)[24] provide an overview of systematic reviews on professional behaviour change interventions. They make an important point that, with the exception of passive dissemination, most interventions are effective under some circumstances but none are effective under all circumstances. Gross *et al.* (2001)[25] say there is general agreement that an integrated multifaceted approach is required to change clinical behaviour on the basis of evidence. As NICE (2002)[26] argues, interventions should consider the barriers to change and use strategies specifically aimed at overcoming them. A summary of the Grimshaw *et al.* (2001)[24] overview was published as part of an effective care bulletin from the NHS Centre for Reviews and Dissemination (1999).[27] It is also available from http://www.york.ac.uk/inst/crd/ech51.pdf.

One problem faced by researchers is the range of development and implementation methodologies. For example, Davies *et al.* (1994)[28] felt that less credibility may be attributed to guidelines developed by local clinicians and that this could be overcome by involving a respected local opinion leader or recognised national expert. In contrast, Thomson *et al.* (1999)[29] reported that a systematic review, including eight randomised controlled trials (RCTs), concluded that using local opinion leaders had mixed results on clinical practice, due in part to inconsistency in the opinion leaders' activities. In an attempt to overcome this problem the Cochrane Effective Practice and Organisation of Care (EPOC) group has developed a taxonomy of interventions. EPOC's website is www.abdn.ac.uk/hsru/epoc/down.hti.

Table 3.1 shows the relationship between EPOC's taxonomy, the evidence base for effectiveness based on international consensus outlined by Gross et al. (2001)[25] and the development approach for care pathways described in Chapter 1 (Figure 1.1). The application of the development and implementation steps for care pathways is consistent with EPOC's taxonomy as it uses a multifaceted approach. The value of care pathways as a vehicle to implement evidence into clinical practice is clearly demonstrated.

Dealing with resistance

There is often some resistance to the care pathway during the processes of development and implementation. Accepting this enables the team to prepare for it and discuss in advance what some of the barriers might be and how they might be overcome.

Very often individuals involved in the development and implementation of pathways will raise practical issues relating to the use of the concept. For example: how can you include the clinical evidence and guidelines without making the care pathway document large and unwieldy? How can you keep the pathway documentation up to date with all the changes/amendments required by the users without frequent and costly printing? Sometimes these objections are simply about the individual trying to understand how they can use the tool in their own working environment. Sometimes they are indicative of a more deep-seated resistance to change and by describing lots of practical problems an individual can create a very effective 'blocking strategy'.

It is essential to determine whether a barrier is resistance or the same goal being looked on from an alternative viewpoint. The barrier needs to be recognised and defined before appropriate action can be taken and this is best achieved by communicating with the resister.

From a practical day-to-day perspective, communication can be described as the effective giving and receiving of a message to an individual or group, involving any medium. It is probably the most important life skill that we have and of its four components – speaking, listening, reading and writing – listening is probably the most underused.

Table 3.1 Relationship between EPOC's taxonomy, the evidence base for effectiveness and the steps identified in the implementation stage of care pathway development

Taxonomy of implementation interventions (EPOC)	Effectiveness evidence base[25]	Care pathway implementation steps
Educational materials – distribution of published or printed recommendations for clinical care, including clinical practice guidelines, audiovisual materials and electronic publications whether delivered personally or through personal or mass mailings.	**Generally ineffective** May raise awareness but seldom change clinical behaviour.	Distribute final draft of care pathway documentation.
Conferences – Participation of healthcare providers in conferences, lectures, workshops or traineeships.	**Generally ineffective** Didactic educational interventions do not appear to change performance. Interactive educational interventions have been shown to effect change.	Awareness raising conference – what is a care pathway and benefits. Interactive training sessions of critiquing sample care pathways. Interactive training at the pre-pilot training sessions of the care pathway involving a review of illustrative patient case history reviews and completion of documentation training.
Local consensus process – inclusion of local providers in discussion to ensure that they agree that the chosen clinical problem is important and that the approach to managing the problem is appropriate. The consensus process may address the design of an intervention to improve performance.	**Variably effective** Can bring together opinion leaders and objectors and effect a change in clinical behaviour.	Use of multi-professional groups to develop the care pathways.

Continued

Table 3.1 Continued

Taxonomy of implementation interventions (EPOC)	Effectiveness evidence base[25]	Care pathway implementation steps
Educational outreach visits – use of a trained person who meets with providers in their practice settings to give information with the intent of changing the provider's performance.	**Generally effective** Most beneficial as 1:1 educational exchange, e.g. information on new drugs, but less effective for other interventions.	Education for staff directly and not directly involved in the pathway.
Local opinion leader – use of providers nominated specifically **by their colleagues** as 'educationally influential'.	**Variably effective**	Support from physicians and hospital leaders – 'local champions'.
Patient-mediated interventions – any intervention aimed at changing the performance of healthcare providers where specific information was sought from or given to patients, e.g. direct mailing to patients, patient counselling delivered by someone other than the targeted providers, educational material given to patients or placed in waiting rooms.	**Variably effective** Consumer education, e.g. providing patients with information about appropriate healthcare interventions has been shown to have a positive effect but is condition dependent.	Patient/user involvement in the development of the individual care pathways. Patient/user access to the care pathway documentation when applied to individual patients.

Audit and feedback – any summary of clinical performance over a period of time. It may include average number of diagnostic tests ordered, average cost per test or per patient, average number per prescriptions written, the proportion of times a desired clinical action was taken etc. The summary may also include recommendations for clinical care. The information may be written or verbal.	**Variably effective** Most effective for prescribing and test ordering.	Compare outcomes to baseline data. Examine variances from care pathway. Communicate results to all involved.
Reminders (manual or computerised) – any intervention that prompts the provider to perform a patient- or encounter-specific clinical action.	**Generally effective** When used sparingly.	Care pathway documentation acts as a template/prompt at the point of care to aid clinical decision making.
Marketing – The use of personal interviewing, group discussion or a survey of targeted providers to identify barriers to change and the subsequent design of an intervention that addresses those barriers.	**Generally effective**	Develop organisational-wide strategy for development and implementation.
Multifaceted interventions – any intervention that includes two or more of the above.	**Generally effective**	Care pathways involve multifaceted interventions.

Table 3.2 Relationship between levels of communication and levels of involvement

Level of involvement	Level of communication	Method of communication
Raise awareness	Give information	Website, newsletter, group brief, notice-boards
Promote understanding	Listen to their views and clarify issues	One to one
Gain their support	Align agendas, find common ground	One to one
Get them involved	Use their creativity and enthusiasm to solve problems	One to one Workshop
Maintain their commitment	Help them to troubleshoot	Project management support

Individuals will have different levels of involvement in the development and implementation of the care pathway. Communication with them should be targeted to meet their needs. Table 3.2 gives an example of how the required level of involvement might affect the level and method of communication.

It is important to bear in mind that the context of a message can affect the way it is interpreted, for example if the same message were sent using electronic mail and face to face, with electronic mail tone of voice and body language can not be conveyed and the message is more likely to be misinterpreted.

If we consider the principal barriers to communication between someone who is tasked with facilitating the development of a care pathway and a practitioner, the list would include some of the following issues (illustrative examples are included):

- gaining access to the other party
- position power
- priority levels (e.g. who decides on the areas in which to develop care pathways – the clinicians, the commissioners, the organisations' management, all of them jointly?)
- misinterpretation of intent (e.g. is the care pathway going to be used to save money, improve quality or both?)

- knowledge levels (e.g. understanding what a care pathway is and its benefits and that it does not restrict the application of professional judgement)
- approach (e.g. pick high-volume, high-cost or complex high-risk conditions)
- time (for development of individual care pathways – meetings/discussions etc.)
- clinical pressures on time
- attitude (e.g. to changes in practice, to care pathways and to multi-professional documentation).

All of these factors might be interpreted as resistance and it is important that we try to understand the viewpoint of the other party.

Covey (1992)[30] said one of the habits of highly effective people is 'seek first to understand'. Covey describes empathic listening as:

> . . . much more than registering, reflecting or even understanding the words that are said. . . . In empathic listening you listen with your ears, but . . . more importantly you listen with your eyes and with your heart. You listen for feeling and for meaning. You listen for behaviour. You use your right brain as well as your left. You sense you intuit you feel.
>
> (pp. 240–1)

You need to clarify the other party's position to the extent that you can label the resistance. Ideally the aim is to find some common ground or, where there is none, to demonstrate that you respect the other person's opinion. You will need to negotiate from this position of understanding and respect but bear in mind that if the other party is prepared to negotiate with you they are also showing a level of commitment to your cause.

Negotiation/consensus building

The *Concise Oxford Dictionary* defines negotiation as 'conferring with others in order to reach a compromise or agreement'.

Consensus building and negotiation sit on a continuum. They offer a very effective process for identifying the needs and interests of parties involved and working towards reconciliation so that both sides can be at least partly satisfied with the result. Both parties are enabled to communicate with one another about objectives, feelings and values, and to bargain.

If someone is prepared to negotiate with you they have a commitment to the cause (those who don't care don't negotiate).

Negotiation and consensus require soft people skills and five of Covey's (1992)[30] seven habits of highly effective people are relevant:

1 First seek to understand – listen, clarify and reflect back what you have heard to demonstrate that you have understood.
2 Choose your response – show respect for their opinions. Consider what you want to convey. Match the non-verbal messages to the words.
3 Keep your core values in mind.
4 Be creative – consider what can you bring to the argument that might help.
5 'Win:win' or no deal.

When, in the perception of those involved, one party gains because of a sacrifice by the other and parties feel that they have mutually incompatible goals, strategies and tactics, the negotiation can easily deteriorate, characterised by secrecy, bluffing and lack of trust.

When both parties realise that they must make sacrifices in order to survive, and the outcome is 'lose:lose', bargaining is generally co-operative due to the overriding goal of survival. A useful source of information and research on negotiation is available at www.batna.com.

This process of consensus building is fundamental to the development of care pathways. If consensus is not reached as to the content of the care pathway by the multidisciplinary team of developers, then it is unlikely to be successfully implemented. If there is a sense that the content of the care pathway has been 'imposed' either on individuals within the development group or from outside, then ownership of the care pathway will not be achieved.

Leadership

The NHS Plan (2000)[31] frequently refers to the need for talented and effective leaders in the NHS. Indeed there is a direct link between good leadership and quality healthcare. Moss and Garside (2001)[32] said effective teams provide high-quality care; effective systems, organisations and teams do not exist without effective leadership. Equally a team developing, implementing or working to a care pathway will require leadership.

The role of a leader in the NHS is defined by the Modernisation Agency (www.modern.nhs.uk) as:

- improving patient care, treatment and experience
- promoting a healthier population
- enhancing the NHS's reputation as a well-managed and accountable organisation
- motivating and developing staff.

Clearly this is not the task of one person or even a small group of people. Leadership happens from within, not from the 'front'. Leaders need to be able to motivate and empower everyone. Morrell and Capparell (2001)[33] argue that you have to 'motivate your staff to be independent. If you have been a good leader, they will have the determination to succeed on their own.'

Good leadership enables people to achieve more than they would have otherwise achieved.

At the 2002 leadership conference, *Mind the Gap*, Alan Milburn, Minister for Health said, 'Leadership is vital to make change happen'. Good leadership enables an organisation to be flexible to both internal and external changes and to learn from its mistakes, i.e. to become a learning organisation.

Themes of leadership for modernisation in the NHS are:

- articulating the vision
- motivation
- decision taking
- releasing talent
- responsiveness and flexibility
- embodying values
- innovative creativity
- working across boundaries
- personal resources.

Many initiatives have been launched to support the development of leadership skills. Going to www.modern.nhs.uk and selecting 'leadership development' will provide more information about the programmes available.

High-quality leadership is essential for successful care pathway development. This leadership is required at a number of levels:

- from the healthcare organisation – to show care pathways are given a high priority within the quality improvement framework of the organisation
- from senior and respected members of the clinical staff within the organisation – Treppel *et al.* (2001)[34] described them as 'champions'
- from the members of the development group – to encourage their colleagues to use the care pathway.

Facilitation

The *Concise Oxford Dictionary* defines facilitation as 'to make easier or more convenient'.

The facilitator works to guide or to smooth a journey to an agreed destination by assisting an individual or group to learn, to solve problems or to generate new ideas. The facilitator supports the use of skills and behaviours to overcome challenges. Facilitation deals with process not with content. The facilitator does not have to be a clinical expert. The role of the facilitator is to ensure a productive process and they may have to act as a leader, a referee or as a neutral observer.

As Johnson (2000),[35] Currie and Harvey (1998)[36] and Middleton and Roberts (2000)[37] point out, facilitation is an essential requirement of care pathway development. Multidisciplinary development groups need someone to act as an unbiased mediator and manage disagreements or conflict within the group. The person needs to be able to ask challenging questions of the group and manage the process of development.

Facilitation can be described as a spectrum ranging from gentle to forceful. As we move along the spectrum the facilitator's behaviour changes from being supportive, through persuasive to being directive. The balance of power between the group being facilitated and the facilitator changes with the group becoming more disempowered as the facilitator becomes more directive. The success of a facilitator is measured by their ability to ensure that the group achieves and retains control.

As a general guide, the facilitator should be trying to work in a supportive way. It is easier for the facilitator to work in this way when:

- there is a mature group with experience
- the aims and objectives are clear
- there is sufficient time
- there is an open, trusting culture/atmosphere
- information is accessible and transparent.

The facilitator should consider all the above points when deciding their approach to the facilitation of the care pathway development. Facilitation is a highly skilled role and a good facilitator will vary their approach according to the group requirements. For example, it is possible to work in a more persuasive – or even directive – way regarding the methodology of development of the care pathway if the group accepts that the facilitator has greater experience and credibility in this area. However, at the same time the facilitator can continue to work in a supportive way, letting the group themselves decide the actual clinical content of the care pathway.

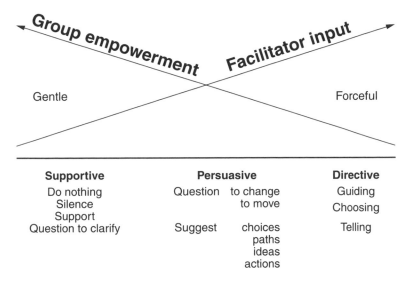

Figure 3.2 Behaviour of facilitator and changes in power base.

Figure 3.2 shows this balance of power diagrammatically and Table 3.3 gives more examples of the type of questions that can be asked relating to the supportive, persuasive and directive approaches.

Sources of assistance

The level of support for organisations involved in developing services is growing almost on a daily basis and inevitably by the time you read this the information will be out of date. However, there are some major sources of support that must be mentioned which will provide a useful starting point in your search for help.

The Modernisation Agency provides support for the NHS in four main areas:

- improving access – helping to provide fast and convenient services
- raising standards of care – improving the quality and standard of the patient experience
- supporting local improvement work – building local capacity for service improvement
- spreading good practice – helping everyone to share their knowledge and learning.

The Modernisation Agency incorporates several teams, for example the National Primary Care Development Team and the Clinical Governance

Table 3.3 Suggested actions for the facilitator

Balance of power	Facilitator behaviour	Suggested facilitator actions	
Group Power	**Supportive**	Do nothing	Sit quietly and do not react in any way to what is happening. Leave the group to work things out for themselves without a hint of whether you agree or disagree, or have any particular feelings about what is happening.
		Silence	Say nothing but express your feelings in body language to influence what is happening.
		Support	Speak or act in such a way that supports what is happening.
		Question to clarify	Provide an opportunity to check that what is happening is what people want to happen. The search for clarity may affect what the group is doing and therefore have an influence.
	Persuasive	Question to change	'Are you ready to go on now?' 'Are you ready to go on yet?'
		Question to move	More specific than changing. Seek to establish the next place the group wants to be: 'OK, so where do you want to go now?' The move on is assumed and emphasis is on where not whether.
		Suggest choices	This action will have direct impact on what the group decides to do next. If you limit the choices you become manipulative.
		Suggest paths	This can affect the balance of the work the group is doing. It is recommended only if the group has lost its way and agreed that they would welcome suggestions on the path to take. It is important to offer a range of paths to allow the group a choice.

	Sharing ideas	This may sound gentle but care must be taken. If the facilitator shares ideas about what is happening the group may see it as an assessment.
	Suggest actions	The most persuasive intervention. For use when the group is completely at a loss what to do next and when the group energy is low. Try to give at least three options.
Directive	Guiding the group	Use when asked or when it is clear that guidance will help the group move forward effectively. The first form of guidance is to suggest what you would do: 'In your situation I would . . .'. The second is to actually do something.
	Choosing for the group	This is leading from the front, choosing what the group will do and where it will go. It should be used rarely and only if requested or if it is perceived that the group is heading for a cliff edge. Recommended intervention would be 'I think it would be useful if we stopped at this point and looked at what is happening. I have a sense we are heading for problems. I would like us to reflect for a moment.' This gives a definite choice to the group.
	Directing	Telling the group what is going to happen next. This form of intervention is the last resort. When all else has failed it may be necessary to direct the group's efforts. The group will react in different ways, some may be relieved, some may be angry and others may cease to participate.

Facilitator Power

Support Team, who between them run many programmes and collaboratives aimed at all levels of healthcare organisations. More information is available on their web page www.modern.nhs.uk.

The collaborative methodology was introduced from the Institute of Healthcare Improvement in Boston, USA and their website www.ihi.org carries additional information and case studies which might be of benefit to the reader.

Further information on the Myers–Briggs type indicator can be found in the following publications:

- Briggs K and Myers I (1987) *Introduction to Type.* Consulting Psychologists Press, Palo Alto, CA.
- Briggs K, Myers I and Myers PB (1980) *Gifts Differing.* Consulting Psychologists Press, Palo Alto, CA.
- Krebs Hirsh S and Kummerow J (1987) *Introduction to Type in Organisational Settings.* Consulting Psychologists Press, Palo Alto, CA.

This chapter has focused on the human aspects of developing and implementing care pathways. In Appendix 3.2, various IT tools and approaches have been listed which may also help with the development process for your care pathways.

Conclusion

To successfully develop, implement and maintain a care pathway within healthcare organisations requires practitioners that are actually going to use the care pathway to:

- own it
- trust it
- believe it will help them deliver improved quality healthcare.

The range of skills, knowledge and experience needed to ensure this happens is extensive. This chapter has attempted to assist the reader in understanding some of these areas and give reference to some sources of help.

References

1 Plamping D (1998) Change and resistance to change in the NHS. *BMJ.* **317**: 69–71. *See also* Plamping D, Gordon P and Pratt J (1998) *Action Zones and Large Numbers.* King's Fund, London.
2 Haines A and Jones R (1994) Implementing findings of research. *BMJ.* **308**: 1488–92.

3 Antman E, Lau J, Kupelnick B, Mosteller F and Chalmers I (1992) A comparison of the results of meta-analysis of randomised controlled trials and recommendations of clinical experts. *JAMA*. **268**: 240–8.

4 Gordon M (1995) Steps to pathway development *Journal of Burn Care and Rehabilitation*. **16**, 197–202.

5 Ahmad F, Bissaker S, de Luc K, Pitts J, Brady S, Dunn L *et al*. (2002) Partnership for developing quality care pathway initiative for people with learning disabilities. Part I: development. *Journal of Integrated Care Pathways*. **6**(1): 9–12.

6 Brady S, Ahmad F, Bissaker S, de Luc K, Pitts J, Dunn L *et al*. (2002) Partnership for developing quality care pathway initiative for people with learning disabilities. Part IIa: hearing impairment. *Journal of Integrated Care Pathways*. **6**(2): 82–5.

7 Pitts J, Ahmad F, Bissaker S, de Luc K, Brady S, Dunn L *et al*. (2002) Partnership for developing quality care pathway initiative for people with learning disabilities. Part IIb: challenging behaviour. *Journal of Integrated Care Pathways*. **6**(2): 86–9.

8 Ahmad F, Bissaker S, de Luc K, Pitts J, Brady S, Dunn L *et al*. (2002) Partnership for developing quality care pathway initiative for people with learning disabilities. Part IIc: epilepsy. *Journal of Integrated Care Pathways*. **6**(2): 90–3.

9 Department of Health (2000) *National Service Framework for Coronary Heart Disease*. DoH, London.

10 Department of Health (2001) *National Service Framework for Older People*. DoH, London.

11 Cameron M and Cranfield S (2001) *Managing Change in the NHS: making informed decisions on change.* NCCSDO, School of Hygiene and Tropical Medicine, London, www.sds.lshtm.ac.uk.

12 Iles V and Sutherland K (2001) *Managing Change in the NHS: organisational change.* NCCSDO, School of Hygiene and Tropical Medicine, London, www.sds.lshtm.ac.uk.

13 Newman K, Payne T and Cowling A (1998) Managing evidence-based healthcare: a diagnostic framework. *Journal of Management in Medicine*. **12**(3): 151–67.

14 Oppenheim AN (1992) *Questionnaire Design, Interviewing and Attitude Measurement*, p. 148. Cassell, London.

15 Jung CG (1971) *Psychological Types*. Princeton University Press, Princeton, NJ. (Originally published as *Psychologische Typen*, 1921.)

16 Myers I and Briggs K (1987) *The Myers–Briggs Type Indicator (MBTI)*. Oxford Psychologists Press, Oxford.

17 West M and Field R (1995) Teamwork in primary healthcare. 1. Perspectives from organisational psychology. *Journal of Interprofessional Care*. **9**(2): 117–22.

18 West MA and Slater JA (1995) Teamwork: myths, realities and research. *Occupational Psychologist*. **24**: 24–9.

19 Guzzo RA and Shea GP (1992) Group performance and inter group relations in organisations. Cited in West MA and Slater JA (1995) Teamwork: myths, realities and research. *Occupational Psychologist*. **24**: 24–9.

20 Firth-Cousins J (1998) Celebrating teamwork. *Quality in Healthcare.* **7**(Suppl): S3–S7.

21 West MA (1994) *Effective Teamwork.* British Psychological Society and Routledge, London. Cited in West MA and Slater JA (1995) Teamwork: myths, realities and research. *Occupational Psychologist.* **24**: 24–9.

22 Batstone G and Edwards M (1996) Achieving clinical effectiveness: just another initiative or a real change in working practice? *Journal of Clinical Effectiveness.* **1**(1): 19–21.

23 Dunning M, Abi-Aad G, Gilbert D, Hutton H and Brouwn C (1998) *Experience, Evidence and Everyday Practice: creating systems for delivering effective healthcare.* Kings Fund, London.

24 Grimshaw J, Shirran L, Thomas R, Mowatt G, Fraser C, Bero L *et al.* (2001) Changing provider behaviour: an overview of systematic reviews of interventions. *Medical Care.* **39**(8).

25 Gross P, Greenfield S, Cretin S, Ferguson J, Grimshaw J, Grol R *et al.* (2001) Optimal methods for guideline implementation. Conclusions from the Leeds Castle meeting. *Medical Care.* **39**(8).

26 National Institute for Clinical Excellence (NICE) (2002) *Principles for Best Practice in Clinical Audit.* Radcliffe Medical Press, Oxford.

27 NHS Centre for Reviews and Dissemination (1999) Getting evidence into practice. *Effective Health Care.* **5**(1).

28 Davies J, Freemantle N, Grimshaw J, Hurwitz B, Long A, Russell I *et al.* (1994) Implementing clinical practice guidelines: can guidelines be used to improve clinical practice? *Effective Health Care.* **8**: 2–11.

29 Thomson MA, Oxman AD, Haynes RB, Davis DA, Freemantle N and Harvey EL (1999) Local opinion leaders to improve health professional practice and healthcare outcomes (Cochrane review). In: *The Cochrane Library*, Issue 1. Update Software, Oxford.

30 Covey SR (1992) *The Seven Habits of Highly Effective People.* Simon & Schuster, London.

31 Secretary of State for Health (2000) *The NHS Plan: a plan for investment, a plan for reform.* The Stationery Office, London. (Cm.4818-I.)

32 Moss F and Garside P (2001) Editorial leadership and learning: building the environment for better, safer healthcare. *Quality in Healthcare.* **10**(2): S1–S2. (www.qualityhealthcare.com)

33 Morrell M and Capparell S (2001) *Shackleton's Way. Leadership lessons from the great Antarctic explorer*, p. 199. Nicholas Brealey, London.

34 Treppel D, Bingham M and Jeffery C (2001) *Getting Started with Integrated Care Pathways.* Health Services Utilisation and Research Commission, Saskatchewan, Canada, http://www.hsurc.sk.ca.

35 Johnson S (2000) Factors influencing the success of ICP projects. *Professional Nurse.* **15**(12): 776–9.

36 Currie L and Harvey G (1998) Care pathways: development and implementation. *Nursing Standard.* **15**(12): 35–8.

37 Middleton S and Roberts A (2000) Getting started. In: Middleton S and Roberts A (eds) *Integrated Care Pathways: a practical approach to implementation*, pp. 38–9. Butterworth-Heinemann, Oxford.

Appendix 3.1: Case study on three different approaches to developing care pathways. Partnership for Developing Quality – West Midlands

Stages of care pathway development	Case study A: Development of four care pathways in learning disabilities	Case study B: Coronary heart disease	Case study C: Stroke care
Choosing the area for the care pathway	Areas chosen: – challenging behaviour – epilepsy – hearing impairment – transitions from child to adult services	Area chosen: chest pain and myocardial infarction	Area chosen: prevention, acute management and rehabilitation of stroke
Ten steps to development[1]			
THE PLANNING PHASE			

1 Development of a project plan – a way forward	Interested parties were invited to a launch day, which included awareness raising and education. They were encouraged to spread their learning and enthusiasm back in their workplaces.
	   It was agreed to develop 'generic' region-wide care pathways in each of the conditions chosen.
		Interested parties were invited to a launch day, which included awareness raising and education.
		   It was agreed to develop a 'generic' region-wide care pathway that could be adapted to suit local organisational environments.
			Interested parties were invited to a launch day which included awareness raising and education. The attendees decided that rather than meet regularly to develop a 'generic' region-wide care pathway which they believed would be too large and onerous to produce, they felt sharing examples of 'good practice' and providing informal support to individuals working in their respective organisations was more important.

Continued

Stages of care pathway development	Case study A: Development of four care pathways in learning disabilities	Case study B: Coronary heart disease	Case study C: Stroke care
• The development groups	Each pathway established a region-wide development group and a steering group was formed to oversee the whole project. All the groups had multidisciplinary, multi-agency membership, which included users.	A region-wide development group was formed with representatives from the multidisciplinary team involved in delivering care for the chest pain/MI patients (including consultant, cardiac nurse, care pathway facilitators, cardiac sister, cardiac rehabilitation co-ordinator and former patients). A steering group was formed to oversee the whole project.	They decided to network and share information electronically. An electronic network was established in 'myworkplace'. More details available on www.nelh.nhs.uk. Each organisation identified a 'lead' to facilitate the development of the care pathway in each of their respective organisations. The group of 'leads' has met on three occasions to share progress and examples of good practice. The work in progress from each organisation can be shared across the region using the electronic network. No steering group was established.
• Facilitation	Separate facilitators who worked in learning disabilities and had an interest in these specific areas facilitated the development groups. Facilitation was 'hands on' with a project manager overseeing all stages. The facilitators had dedicated time allocated to the project. This enabled them to drive the project.	The region-wide group had an external facilitator who was a former cardiac nurse. This person had dedicated time allocated to the project. This person 'drove' the project.	No region-wide facilitator allocated.

2 Background information on the evidence to inform the content			
• Identification of clinical evidence	A literature review found very little research evidence in existence with the exception of epilepsy where there were national evidence-based standards. Current practice from organisations across the region was used as the starting point for discussion.	There was a large body of evidence concerning the management of these patients (including a NSF). However, there was a lack of consensus on the validity of the evidence. The Regional Library Unit undertook to validate the evidence base and found it sound. From this point ownership of the care pathway became easier.	There was a large body of evidence within the NSF. Literature lists relating to stroke care and the use of care pathways were made available electronically to the members of the group.
• Identification of relevant legislation	In the 'transitions' care pathway they identified 22 relevant pieces of legislation that had to be met.		
• Sharing examples of other care pathways	Very few examples of other care pathways within the field of learning disabilities were found. This meant the development groups had to discuss how the concept needed to be adapted to suit their client groups.	It was known that a number of organisations in the region had already done some work in this area so it was decided to undertake a region-wide trawl to identify the work and to avoid 're-inventing the wheel'. The work identified was categorised into four groups using an appraisal tool developed locally:[2] group 1 – no formalised care pathway group 2 – no pathway but comprehensive data collection system	Sharing experience and learning across teams and organisations is an important aspect of feedback. However, some workgroup members had the perception that their organisations would not 'allow' the sharing of a pathway between organisations even though the patient journey clearly transcended these boundaries.

Continued

Stages of care pathway development	Case study A: Development of four care pathways in learning disabilities	Case study B: Coronary heart disease	Case study C: Stroke care
		group 3 – pathway by name and redesign work taken place group 4 – comprehensive care pathway. A workshop was held to feed back the results of the regional trawl to interested parties.	All of the leads felt strongly that the stroke care pathway must cover the entire patient journey to be of real value, i.e. all aspects of care – prevention, acute management and rehabilitation. Work continues in all these areas.

THE DEVELOPMENT PHASE

3 Scope the care pathway (beginning and end)	Identification of the group of clients to be included in the pathway was easier for some pathways than others. The challenging behaviour group took a long time to narrow down its scope from covering all aspects of challenging behaviour to a 'crisis situation'.	Other examples of cardiac pathways were used to scope the care pathway and a decision was taken to start the pathway once the patient reached the hospital (A&E or CCU). Later in the project one of the ambulance services approached the development group asking for the pathway to be extended to cover their service (this phase remains work in progress).	

4 Process map the care	Each development group designed an 'ideal process map' with standards and attached it to the pathway documentation.	Each organisation was asked to map out the services currently provided in each organisation and to identify the differences from the process being outlined in the 'generic' care pathway documentation.	Each organisation was asked to map out the services currently provided in each organisation and to identify the differences from the process being outlined in the 'generic' care pathway documentation.
5 Design the care pathway documentation	The pathway documents replace existing clinical documentation and requires the nomination of a care co-ordinator for each client put on the pathway. The documentation is multi-disciplinary. In the 'transitions' pathway two documents are being developed. The main pathway document is planned to be held by the client and designed in pictorial/easy-to-understand format. The practitioners will hold a check-list of tasks/goals and further information.	A 'generic' region-wide pathway document was developed which identified different stages in the pathway and the goals.	Each organisation is developing its own documentation to support the use of the care pathway.

THE IMPLEMENTATION PHASE

6 Plan the changes	Each care pathway had the new standards included within the care pathway identified along with the changes required to achieve the standards (i.e. a gap analysis).	Each site was encouraged to adapt the tool to suit local circumstances.	Care pathways still in development phase.

Continued

Stages of care pathway development	Case study A: Development of four care pathways in learning disabilities	Case study B: Coronary heart disease	Case study C: Stroke care
7 Train the staff	The facilitators visited all the pilot sites to discuss the project and train staff.	Three training workshops were held around the region for interested parties to discuss the content of the pathway and decide whether they wanted to pilot.	All interested parties were offered a training session to use the electronic 'virtual community' system.
8 Pilot (test) the pathway	Three of the care pathways have been piloted in between two and four sites each across the region and the transitions care pathway is due to be piloted shortly. A lead in each pilot site was identified to feed back progress/issues problems and to undertake additional training.	The pathway has been adapted and is being piloted (or due to be) in four sites across the region.	
9 Sign off the care pathways	The piloted pathways have been evaluated externally. The results of the evaluation and impact of the care pathway on staff and users have been reported at a conference. Planning for the roll-out of the three completed care pathways for any organisations wishing to be involved is progressing. The transitions pathway is still in development.	One of the pilot sites has approved the care pathway for permanent use. The other three sites are still to do so.	

10 Maintenance and update

Work ongoing.

Work ongoing.

TIMESCALE FOR DEVELOPMENT

from launch to pilot phase

December 2000–June 2002 (work still in progress for the transitions pathway)

November 2000–ongoing

January 2002–ongoing

[1] de Luc K (2002) The ten-step guide to developing a care pathway. *Nurse 2 Nurse.* **2**(10): 10–12.
[2] de Luc K and Whittle C (2002) An integrated care pathway appraisal tool – a badge of quality. *Journal of Integrated Care Pathways.* **6**: 13–17.

Appendix 3.2: Sources of assistance using computer software

This appendix provides some examples of how computer software can support care pathway development and implementation. The objective is to raise awareness of the potential and encourage experimentation, rather than to provide a specific 'tool kit'. Local IT infrastructure and standards, access to IT equipment and the IT skills of team members and facilitators will have a significant influence on what is possible and worthwhile. The emphasis is on IT tools for individuals, teams and local organisations. Broader issues of national standards and enabling infrastructure are covered in Chapters 6 and 7. We cannot, however, see how a clear line can be drawn between local and national infrastructure and initiatives – they are interdependent.

Where specific manufacturers or products are mentioned, we are not providing recommendations or endorsements, but merely citing typical examples and software features. Readers are strongly recommended to consult their local IT services department to check compatibility and training needs before purchase.

In the UK during the 1990s, care pathway development teams have, in general, had access to minimal IT tools. Typically, word-processing soft-ware would be used like an electronic typewriter to generate unstructured documents, with manual annotation and transcription of changes. Word processor functions would also be used more or less effectively to design forms and to draw simple process maps and flow charts – usually without reference to defined diagramming standards. Electronic mail (e-mail) might be used as a rapid postal service to deliver word processor files to team members, who may have kept local personal copies or printed versions in paper files.

As we look forward to development of computerised care pathways over the next decade, we believe more sophisticated use of IT tools and information sources is both possible and desirable, specifically:

- development and maintenance of care pathways in a structured form
- improved diagramming, documentation and presentation
- high-speed access to local intranets and the Internet for file sharing and access to evidence
- management at a personal and team/speciality level of evidence sources
- development of 'online communities'
- improved dialogue with IT staff for implementation of computerised care pathways
- improved access to statistical data on activity, outcomes, clinical incidents, workforce etc. to support whole-community change using care pathways.

Examples of more sophisticated use of software tools include the following:

- Specialist evidence management software is already available, but is generally for personal use.[1,2] However, there is a trend towards more community-wide evidence management using innovative combinations of local software and Internet capabilities.[3]
- Once a care pathway is developed in a structured form it can be output in several different formats, including word processor file format for output on paper if required.
- Drawing software such as *Microsoft Visio* provides a range of standard diagram types and features, such as linking of lines to shapes so that lines are automatically re-routed if the shape is moved. In the context of this book, simple diagramming software is not recommended for process mapping (*see* Chapter 5), but drawing software is useful during care pathway conceptual development for, e.g. fishbone diagrams, 'mind maps', decision charts etc. Drawings can be readily copied into document files, or converted for publication on intranets.
- Modern word-processing software includes some little-used features that can significantly improve the efficiency and quality of complex shared documents, such as guidelines and care pathways. For example:
  - use of style definitions and style sheets/templates can provide organisation-wide standards for document structure and appearance, which represent local best practice
  - table design features can improve the appearance and usability of forms
  - macros can automate and thus save time spent on common tasks, such as insertion of a standard tick-box. Macros can be embedded in templates so they can be easily shared
  - document management features – ranging from simply including filename and version information automatically in page footers, through to sophisticated version control and cataloguing information in the file header to aid electronic filing and retrieval
  - document reviewing features allow comments and changes by various contributors to be easily tracked and managed by the main author
  - documents can be saved in formats which are suitable for publication on intranets, and which maintain internal structure. Such files are normally 'read only' to maintain version and content control
  - specialist spell-checkers can be obtained for common word processing software which facilitates the checking of the clinical terminology used in care pathways.

- The document publication standard and software known as *Adobe Acrobat* allows files produced in many different formats to be published electronically, with a range of controls over what end-users can see and do. The main benefit is that, provided users have the free *Acrobat Reader* software, they can view and print the document exactly as intended by the author. Many *Acrobat* files (otherwise known as 'pdf' – portable document format) are on the accompanying CD. *Acrobat* files can be accessed directly from within web browser software (such as *Microsoft Internet Explorer*). *Acrobat* format is therefore a better distribution medium than 'native' word processor files, which inevitably cause compatibility problems and the risk of modification of 'master files'.
- Presentation software such as *Microsoft PowerPoint*, or more sophisticated multimedia development software such as *Macromedia Director*, allow facilitators and other specialists to efficiently produce high-quality training materials. These can be used in face-to-face presentations or accessed online via web browsers.
- Project-planning software such as *Microsoft Project* provides facilities to track the roles, tasks, deadlines, deliverables etc. which make up any project. Although probably not worthwhile within single development teams, at an organisation level, or for a care pathway facilitator with several teams running in parallel, project-planning software can provide a useful means of managing complexity and supporting standards.

The main features and uses of software which supports 'on-line communities' are outlined below. Such software provides a new medium for human interaction which is known generally as computer-supported cooperative work (CSCW). CSCW systems cannot substitute for face-to-face meetings, but if managed and supported effectively, CSCW can reduce the frequency and duration of meetings and allow people to participate in groups at times convenient to them. CSCW is especially useful for communities which are widely distributed geographically.

Core CSCW features include:

- e-mail – both simple interpersonal mail, plus distribution lists (personal or shared) and automated mail list servers. The latter relay a message sent to a single address to many recipients who have 'joined' the list by sending a simple sign-on message
- intranets, which may be accessible to staff within one organisation or shared amongst several. Intranets can provide widely varying levels of sophistication, from a simple repository of reference information, through to a platform for many CSCW functions. Typically, intranets would allow individuals to store draft or final documents for others to share

- document management systems, which provide more sophisticated file sharing than a typical intranet, such as version control, search and retrieval, access control
- on-line discussions or 'computer conferencing', which allow members of a topic or 'thread' to add comments and view others' comments.[4-6] Topics might be open or closed (private) and may or may not be moderated. The public domain Internet newsgroups and chat forums are basic examples, but much more sophisticated software exists.[7]

A related term to CSCW, first coined by Wenger, is the 'Community of Practice' (CoP),[8,9] which has influenced a wide range of systems-based approaches including the learning organisation and knowledge management (KM). In KM theory, a Community of Practice usually describes a group with a common (professional) interest working in an environment which encourages sharing of information. Organisational support for CoPs is a critical success factor in KM. Table 3A2.1 below summarises the characteristics of CoPs, as perceived by the Xerox Corporation.[10]

Many of the behaviours shown in the right-hand column in Table 3A2.1 are already demonstrated by the care pathway community at local and regional level. It therefore seems reasonable to assume that if improved supporting IT infrastructure was developed, then care pathway

Table 3A2.1 Main characteristics of communities of practice

CoP characteristic	Actions/consequences
Interaction format	Meetings, collaborative computing, interaction structure, e-mail etc.
Organisational culture	Leverages common training, experience and vocabulary. Facilitates working around constraints
Mutual interest	Builds commitment and promotes continuous improvement of processes
Individual and collective learning	Recognises and rewards knowledge contribution and use; leverages knowledge; provides a culture of knowledge sharing
Knowledge sharing	Embeds knowledge sharing into work practices. Reinforces with immediate feedback the value of knowledge sharing
Community processes and norms	Build trust and identity. Minimise linkage to formal control structure. Motivate the community to establish its own governance processes

developers would make immediate use of it without a significant 'culture shift'. This theme is developed further in Chapter 7.

At a purely local level, those facilitating the development of care pathways and working with IT and information management staff have a clear leadership role in improving the use of IT tools to support care pathway development. For example, general IT awareness and specific software skills will increasingly become a basic competency for clinical staff and therefore need to be included in staff appraisal schemes and personal development plans.

A final 'health warning' is called for – much of the IT support for care pathways involves accessing the Internet. From an information security point of view, the Internet is a very hostile place. All staff accessing the Internet, whether from work, home or university campus, should be protected by up-to-date anti-virus software.

References

1 Booth A (2000) Organising a personal knowledge base. In: A Booth (ed.) *Managing Knowledge in Health Services*. Library Association Publishing, London.
2 ISI Research Soft Product Comparison, http://www.researchsoft.com/rscompare.asp.
3 Booth A (2000) Keeping up to date with the knowledge base. In: A Booth (ed.) *Managing Knowledge in Health Services*. Library Association Publishing, London.
4 Hiltz SR and Turoff M (1993) *The Network Nation* (revised edition). MIT Press, Cambridge, MA. (http://eies.njit.edu/~turoff)
5 Dix AJ (1994) Computer-supported cooperative work – a framework. In: D Rosenburg and C Hutchison (eds) *Design Issues in CSCW*. Springer Verlag, Heidelberg. (*See* CD.)
6 Winograd T (1987) A language/action perspective on the design of cooperative work. *Human-Computer Interaction*. **3**(1): 3–30. (http://hci.stanford.edu/~winograd/papers/language-action.html) (*See* CD.)
7 http://www.smartgroups.com
8 Wenger E (1998) *Communities of Practice: learning, meaning and identity*. Cambridge University Press, New York. (http://www.ewenger.com/)
9 http://www.cpsquare.com
10 Adapted from Storck J and Hill PA (2000) Knowledge diffusion through strategic communities. *Sloan Management Review*. **41**(2). Reprinted in Turban E *et al*. (2002) *Information Technology for Management* (3e). John Wiley, New York.

Building a computerised care pathway: practical lessons

Margaret Craddock

Key points

- The computerisation of a paper-based care pathway aids informed clinical decision making in the management of individual patients.

- Computerised care pathways are qualitatively different from paper-based pathways. They enable new ways of working which are not possible in a paper-based environment.

- It is essential that care pathway development teams are fully engaged in service commissioning in their local health community to ensure that the new ways of working which become possible are reflected in service planning and resource allocation.

Introduction

This chapter describes the issues arising from converting an established paper-based care pathway into a computerised version which will form part of the electronic patient record (EPR). The logistics of conversion are demonstrated from the clinician's perspective. The focus of the work reported here is on redesign of evidence-based care processes by taking advantage of the benefits of clinical computer systems.

Background

As part of the modernisation of the UK National Health Service, the Government has set out an information strategy entitled *Information for Health: an information strategy for the modern NHS 1998–2005* (1998).[1] This document, plus more recent updates,[2] sets out a timetable and targets for the implementation of information technology to directly support patient care. The opportunity now exists to align and co-ordinate the development of both clinical practice and information management.

Contained within the national information strategy were a number of initiatives, one of which includes the development of an electronic health record (EHR). The aim of the EHR is to provide summarised key clinical information about a patient, ultimately 'from the cradle to the grave'. A second initiative was to develop an EPR. The differences between the two concepts need clarifying. In addition to relevant demographic details and clinical history, the EPR contains detailed clinical information about the care provided for a specific patient. The information strategy identified several levels of EPR implementation, where the higher levels aimed to achieve the ultimate goal of a fully electronic record, accessible at any time and tailored to the needs of the particular healthcare professional. Even at basic levels of implementation, an EPR should support evidence-based care and standards for disease management, e.g. coronary heart disease and stroke. The EPR should also have the potential to hold these clinical details irrespective of where that care is delivered, i.e. primary, secondary or social care. If the care is provided against a pre-defined plan, this is effectively the computerised care pathway.

In contrast, the EHR focuses on providing key summaries from EPRs which provide core information about a patient, e.g. demographics, immunisation status, which care pathway they are enrolled in, outcomes of previous contacts with health services etc.

The case study: stroke services in Walsall

Walsall is situated in the West Midlands, or the central region of England, and has an estimated population of 260 900 people. It is an area of great diversity in the distribution of young and old, ethnicity, culture and income. It contains some of the most deprived wards in the country, and others of some affluence. Historically, Walsall has had the highest morbidity and mortality rates for coronary heart disease and stroke in the West Midlands.

Walsall has an integrated stroke service that spans two NHS trusts – one trust covers the acute hospital services, the other is a primary care trust that includes general practitioners and community health services. The integrated stroke service also interfaces with social services in the borough of Walsall. This case study outlines the work of the stroke team to clearly define and document the stroke care pathway, ensuring the contents are evidence-based, patient-focused and assist transfer of care across organisations. The main focus of this case study has been to convert an already existing paper-based care pathway into a computerised one that provides health and social care professionals with:

- accurate, complete and immediately available information about individual patients
- access to guidelines and knowledge to support clinical decision making
- access to information to evaluate their clinical effectiveness and support continuing education.

To achieve these goals, the clinical team depended on the expertise provided by the local IT services department to support the clinicians and to provide education and training and advice on security and confidentiality issues. Because the IT developments in Walsall were novel in several respects (at least in the UK), direct support from the software supplier was also important.

How the stroke care pathway fits into the current UK health agenda

In developing our stroke care pathway, the clinical team were responding to a number of external and internal drivers. The external drivers were:

- *A First Class Service* (1998)[3] discusses quality and clinical effectiveness, and refers to the care pathway as an appropriate tool to deliver this objective.
- The Royal College of Physicians (RCP) *Sentinel Audit* (2000)[4] supports benchmarking and an opportunity for clinicians to measure their performance against national data, thus enabling them to improve quality of care.
- The RCP *National Clinical Guidelines for Stroke* (1999)[5] is a robust document which provides clinicians and commissioners in all settings with a sound evidence base and targets to appropriately manage stroke patients.
- The *National Service Framework For Older People* (2001)[6] specified rather ambitious milestones and timescales. One of its aims was to reduce the incidence of stroke in the population and ensure that those who have had a stroke have prompt access to integrated stroke care services. Standard Five states that:

> The NHS will take action to prevent strokes, working in partnership with other agencies where appropriate. People who are thought to have had a stroke have access to diagnostic services, are treated appropriately by specialist stroke service, and subsequently, with their carers, participate in a multidisciplinary programme of secondary prevention and rehabilitation.

The milestone is that 100% of all general hospitals which care for people with stroke should have a specialised stroke service by April 2004. The stroke team harnessed the opportunity to use the four key components of stroke management contained within the document – prevention, immediate care, early and continuing rehabilitation and long-term support – to extend their existing paper-based stroke care pathway.

The internal drivers were that the organisations involved in developing the computerised stroke care pathway believe that:

- care pathways provide a mechanism to ensure best practice and that they facilitate a process of care/treatment which can be monitored, reviewed and evaluated
- the care pathway ensures completion of the audit loop by identifying and collecting variances from the expected care pathway, which ultimately objectively and positively demonstrates gaps in service provision
- clinical risk management is improved as best practice is identified throughout the care pathway.

Constructing the computerised care pathway

The paper-based stroke care pathway has been running for approximately four years, and has involved up to 70 care professionals and service managers. The maturity of the team and the paper-based care pathway was one of the reasons for identifying stroke as the computerised care pathway pilot. The stroke team had already seen considerable benefits from the original project to develop a paper-based care pathway. These included:

- The measurement and clear understanding by all the team of what was happening to patients who used their services pre-pathway. A baseline audit of services was completed to demonstrate the changes before and after implementation.
- The current and the future direction of the service was identified through mapping the patient journey at a high level. It was at this stage (April 2001) that the stroke team recognised the potential to include the four key interventions (prevention, immediate care, early and continuing rehabilitation and long-term support) outlined in the *National Service Framework for Older People*.
- The care pathway was clearly supporting the existing shared record of care by maximising collaboration between teams, disciplines and organisations. Debates focused on which interventions were to be performed by which discipline, and when. Clinical protocols and measurable outcomes were designed which enabled data and variances to be collected and analysed. For example, following assessment, therapists were able to estimate the number of treatment sessions per week a patient may require to promote rehabilitation potential and achieve predicted outcomes. When clinicians were unable to deliver treatments, for whatever reason, this was recorded as a variance. Anecdotally, staff had raised concerns about low staffing levels previously, now there was a mechanism to objectively demonstrate gaps in therapy provision.
- Redefining the care pathway enabled patients' individual needs to be incorporated and clinical judgement to be utilised, thus preventing the pathway from becoming a simple check-list of tasks.
- Greater equity of care was achieved for all patients, regardless of their geographical location within the local healthcare system.
- There was an enhancement of the team dynamics. 'Tribalism' reduced dramatically both within disciplines and across the primary and acute care providers. Duplication of clinical records across these organisations was reduced as a result of a greater level of trust and understanding of each other's role.

- Building in a robust audit trail was particularly important to the stroke team. In addition to guiding clinicians through an episode of care, it proved invaluable in demonstrating gaps in service provision and was an effective tool to inform the health and social care commissioning process.

So by the end of 2001 the stroke team had defined the information requirements to deliver stroke care, and had used a paper-based care pathway document for four years. There was now a strong drive from clinicians for shared access to data from each organisation involved in patient care, presented in a logical, seamless and accessible format – in other words, the team now required the technology to support the integrated way of working they had devised on the paper-based care pathway.

The IT requirement

The technical infrastructure to develop computerised care pathways has been available (in its broadest sense) in the IT marketplace for a considerable length of time. However, in the UK health service, IT systems across both acute and primary care have historically been mainly administration and management systems, used to track patients around wards and clinics, with aggregated data on activity extracted to support service planning and funding. They have not, in the main, focused on supporting the provision of clinical services to patients. However, at Walsall, clinical computing provision in the acute sector was higher than average. Clinicians could access computerised radiology and pathology results, with intranet and Internet access to clinical guidelines and protocols. Within primary care, whilst clinicians could also access investigation results, the process was cumbersome, requiring the user to log in/out of various systems. The information regarding a patient's disease management whilst hospitalised, and ongoing clinical management within primary care, sat in different IT systems. Social care records were separate again. The overall picture was one of 'islands of computerisation' separated by a variety of networks, including traditional postal services, faxes and telephone calls.

What the stroke team required was a system that allowed for collection of and access to all patient-specific details, from the point of onset of condition, to discharge, to follow-up, which would facilitate a seamless transfer of care. In essence, an integrated system which would provide:

- elimination of multiple log-ins and one secure central log-in
- one patient search across all systems using a single patient identifier (the NHS number)
- simple access to multiple clinical applications, e.g. imaging, pathology results.

Development of the stroke computerised care pathway became part of a programme of work to implement improved clinical computing. At the time of writing, most of the IT infrastructure is in place and the stroke computerised care pathway is undergoing final acceptance testing.

The new IT infrastructure does not in general replace existing systems, but instead integrates patient data held in multiple clinical and administrative systems into a unified view. However, the new system can itself hold data about patients if there is no existing system to 'fill the gap'. The new system also acts as a 'message centre', generating and relaying messages between other computers and between care professionals. The type of data which is displayed and the way it is presented can be tailored to the needs of particular types of user. Because the new system is accessed via normal web browser software, it can still function adequately over slow data communications links. For example, community-based stroke follow-up nurses can access and update patient records from a patient's home via their own telephone line or a mobile data link. Consequently the speed, accuracy, reliability and security of communication between care professionals has improved significantly.

The scope of the computerised stroke care pathway

The stroke team decided that only the 'stroke follow-up' stage of the existing paper-based care pathway should be computerised first, as a proof of concept (*see* Figure 4.1).[7] The reasons for choosing stroke follow-up were:

- the acute stroke pathway follows predominately a medical model and would therefore not engage all multidisciplinary team members
- there was a robust, co-ordinated stroke follow-up team with excellent communication between members
- this component was active and in practical use by all stroke team members
- it was believed that the proof of concept (by doing the stroke follow-up phase) would generate confidence that the acute stroke phase which spans a time frame of seven days, the rehabilitation phase which is rather more complex to predict, and a prevention pathway could ultimately be 'bolted on' to provide a whole stroke journey.

The subgroup working on the computerising of the stroke follow-up care pathway included the following people:

- stroke co-ordinator
- stroke liaison nurses
- physiotherapist

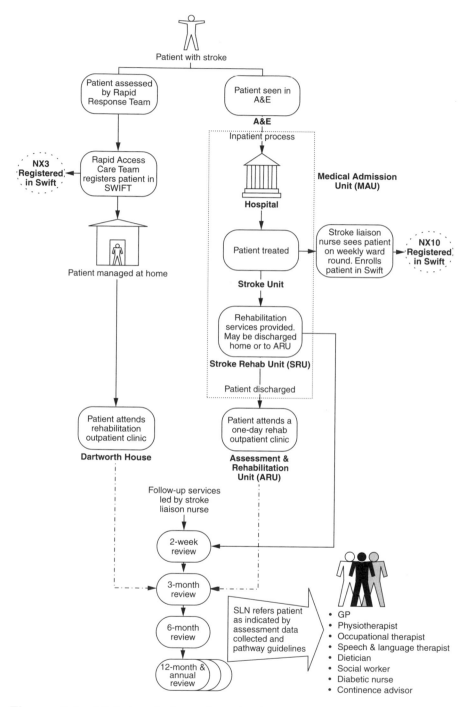

Figure 4.1 High-level view of stroke follow-up within overall stroke pathway.[7]

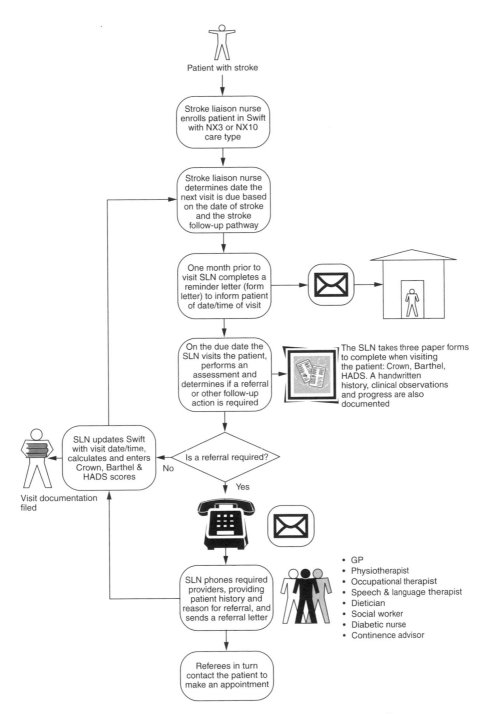

Figure 4.2 Current stroke follow-up process flow.

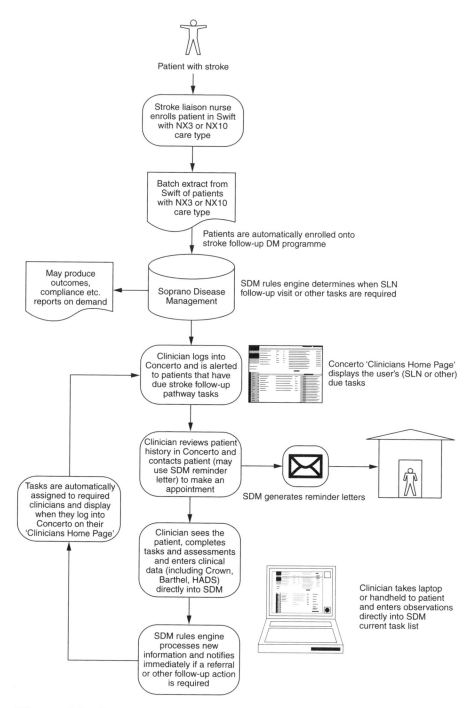

Figure 4.3 Proposed computerised stroke follow-up process flow.

- occupational therapist (OT)
- general practitioner (GP)
- clerk
- healthcare assistant.

Process flow for the patient

Figures 4.2 and 4.3 show respectively the paper-based and electronic process flows for stroke follow-up. In the paper-based process flow, all patients with a diagnosis of stroke are entered onto a stroke register. Following discharge from hospital, the stroke liaison nurse (SLN) arranges visits to ensure the patient is reassessed at two weeks post-discharge, and then at three months, six months, 12 months and annually from the stroke thereafter. If the patient experiences a subsequent stroke, these visits are rescheduled from the date of the last stroke.

Problems for the clinicians with the paper-based process included:

1 The manual system depended on the SLN being informed by telephone/fax/letter of all stroke patients. There was always the risk of patients being missed.
2 The SLN determined when the next visit was required. This could be a manually intensive task which requires the nurse to access notes to look up case histories.
3 Approximately 250 appointment letters per month were generated by hand, which was time-consuming.
4 During a patient visit, significant clinical detail was recorded by the SLN. The assessment tool used scores calculated using Barthel and Crown II schemes to determine new clinical deficits, which in turn determine referral requirements. (Barthel is a validated functional assessment tool to indicate levels of dependence/independence in activities of daily living. In Walsall, another extended tool called Crown II is also used locally for the same purposes.)[8] In the manual system, the scores for both these tools were calculated manually and any subsequent referrals were also produced manually. The data was collected on paper and subsequently re-keyed into a patient administration system by administrative staff. The clinical record of the assessment did not therefore form part of a clinical work-flow system and there was no means of tracking progress against referral and care plan decisions.
5 If the patient needed to re-enter rehabilitation services, the SLN has to refer to the stroke team within primary care. These clinicians had only limited access to the recent patient history; therefore a summary had to be provided manually by the referring clinician.

6 Should a patient have a new stroke, clinicians in secondary care, or from other services, could experience delays and/or incomplete information sharing. This was potentially a clinical risk.

7 Performing paper-based clinical audits to determine adherence to the pathway was extremely time-consuming. It may not be immediately apparent what has or has not been done and whether local or national quality standards have been achieved.

Through the implementation of a stroke computerised care pathway, many of the manual activities are automated and the issues summarised above are addressed thus:

1 There is automated enrolment onto the stroke care pathway. This means it is not possible to miss any patients.

2 All clinicians have equal access to the patient record to review clinical history, which will support their decision making and avoid duplication of data capture. This avoids unnecessary questions to the patients, reduces dependency on the patient (or their carers) to mediate the transfer of care between agencies/professions and generally improves the accuracy and completeness of records.

3 The stroke computerised care pathway automates appointment letters, thereby saving clinicians' time. Information captured is entered electronically and directly into the system, immediately calculating risk scores by responding to the 'rules' (see below) which have been created within the system and displayed as drop down menus for the clinician to choose from, for example evidence-based range statements for cholesterol levels or units of alcohol consumed. The clinician selects an option, which supports their decision making, and electronically identifies a new task to be completed, for example 'refer to the GP for review of medication'.

4 If a referral is required, a task reminder is automatically generated for that clinician, and they will have immediate access to review the clinical history. The SLN is saved the time-consuming task of writing referral letters and following up with other clinicians.

5 Should the patient have subsequent stroke events, clinicians in secondary care have immediate access to view potentially important history.

6 Clinical audits can be performed by defining reports from the system, and can be linked to evidence-based practice standards.

7 Users can directly access summaries or full text of relevant clinical evidence from within an individual patient record.

8 Users can override the default actions suggested by the computerised care pathway and record the reason for their decision. Coupled with the improved reporting system, this allows better monitoring of variances

and supports regular review/development of the computerised care pathway.

Creating rules and tasks

Using best practice guidelines and clinical evidence, sets of 'rules' and 'tasks' were created. The rules represent, in computerised form, the 'decision trees' which are commonly found in clinical guidelines and protocols, plus other local agreements about flow of work between professionals within the stroke team. The tasks may include treatments, checks or investigations to be carried out, data items and observations to be captured. These are put into action according to the rules relating to certain data, e.g. lifestyle factors, performance measures, blood pressure ranges, weight, smoking/drinking habits etc.

For example, in the assessment section of the previous paper version of the care pathway there was a section on smoking history. Once this information had been collected by the clinician it was passed to a clerk and entered into the community patient contact management system. The data were held mainly as a historic record and did not directly affect the clinical work-flow for the individual patient. The actual data on a given patient's smoking habits might or might not generate a referral to the smoking cessation team, due to operational and communications obstacles to efficient work-flow.

In the electronic equivalent, the team had to research the evidence base for smoking cessation counselling as a therapeutic input and then build the rule set which automatically produced the referral if certain conditions were met. Clearly, changes in clinical work-flow which are enabled by the computerised care pathway had to be agreed by all stakeholders and properly resourced. Similar development work was replicated in many different parts of the stroke follow-up care pathway. Appendix 4.1 shows example screen shots of the user's view of the system.

Time to develop

Overall, the team have taken approximately one year to develop the working computerised system. This includes identifying the rules, evidence base, data entry forms, user interface, messages, test plans, documentation, training plans and materials, security controls, system design and configuration. In total, the net effort by the project co-ordinator, clinical staff and IT staff involved in the pilot has been estimated as approximately one person year.

This may seem like a long time and a significant effort. However, this was a new undertaking for all concerned, which added to the time and effort required. Given the overall state of NHS clinical computing, the project should be regarded as research and development rather than a conventional IT system implementation. Also, in general, clinical staff were working on the project in addition to their normal duties.

Future computerised care pathway development and implementation projects are expected to take less time and resource, but it is clear from the stroke follow-up pilot that the potential benefits of computerised care pathways can only be achieved at a price in terms of additional clinical team effort. This case study has identified a number of issues which need to be addressed if successful development and implementation of computerised care pathways are to be achieved.

Lessons learnt

The computerised care pathway is not simply a computerised version of the paper-based care pathway. Rather, the efficiencies provided by the computerised system enable improved ways of working to be introduced for a given level of service funding. Thinking through the precise detail of decision trees in effect promoted the development of a new version of the stroke follow-up care pathway. This new version:

- is more evidence-based
- includes a richer set of options, for example the pathway can now focus clinicians' time on modifiable risk factors and secondary prevention
- has moved away from collecting clinical data for administrative and management purposes to aiding informed clinical decision making in the management of individual patients
- has improved teamworking, for example clinicians across acute and community services now actively share lessons learnt in anticipation of working together on developing the next phase of the computerised stroke care pathway.

The computerised version of the stroke care pathway represents a more optimum model of care. This improvement process can be related to two of the four 'killer Bs' identified by Sackett *et al.* (2000)[9] and described in Chapter 2. Computerised care pathways provide more efficient and reliable communications and enable new ways of working, which affects the local resource **bargain** and removes some of the **barriers** to implementing evidence-based practice.

Essential requirements for successful development and implementation include:

- An understanding and acceptance by the clinical team of work-flow and messaging concepts and their potential benefits.
- Clinical staff need to specify in rigorous detail, in a form suitable for computerisation, the tasks and rules which govern the individual patient journey.
- Overall usability and the overhead of staff training can be significantly affected by the design of the human–computer interface. Sequences of computer screens and the electronic forms which support data entry and display are more complex than paper-based forms.
- New team structures which include IT, information and perhaps also clinical audit staff are required to develop computerised care pathways.
- As well as piloting the clinical aspects of the pathway, computerised care pathway implementations require thorough testing of the software and the new work-flow.
- Computerised care pathway development teams will increasingly have to incorporate nationally mandated data sets, designed to ensure that consistent information is available to support comparative audit of practice and outcomes.
- There is a need for a culture change amongst clinical staff which promotes the importance of high-quality information to support high-quality care. This can only be achieved when there is a belief that the data coming from the computerised system are reliable and accurate.
- A well thought out and robust security model, supported by system security controls, policies and procedures, is needed. The advantages of flexibility, speed and accessibility of data that computerised care pathways give a health community raise many issue of patient data confidentiality.

Based on the experience of the stroke care pathway team and several others, including coronary heart disease, diabetes, incontinence and rectal bleeding, the Walsall health community is developing an assessment tool to gauge the 'state of readiness' of any team or topic. The key headings included in the tool kit are:

- culture
- multidisciplinary working
- data quality.

In some situations and specialities, the EPR system has been deployed as an improved way of capturing and sharing clinical information as a precursor to full care pathway implementation. In this way the clinical staff involved gain immediate benefits. They also get used to the system and become aware of other potential uses, including care pathways, so

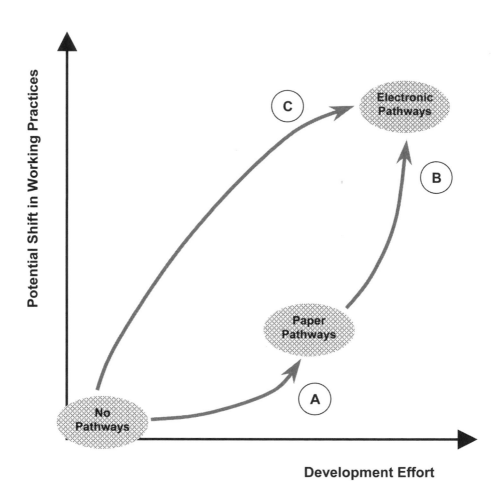

Arrow 'A' represents the conventional care pathway development process.

Arrow 'B' represents the process described in the Walsall case study, where a mature care pathway team took on the additional development and implementation complexity of a computerised care pathway. The benefits of computerisation of patient records and parts of the care process, identified in Chapter 1 and Chapter 4, create opportunities for significantly different ways of working. These may require changes in professional relationships and work patterns, which in turn need shifts in financial resources around a health / social care community.

Arrow 'C' represents the challenge facing most health care communities in order to meet NHS strategic objectives. Change on the scale and at the rate envisaged will require new approaches for individual care pathway teams, whole communities and national agencies and networks.

Figure 4.4 Transitions to computerised care pathways – schematic.

that applications of the system grow more as a process of 'cultural diffusion' than as a conventional centralised IT project.

Because computerised care pathways enable new ways of working, the difference between old and new working practices is likely to be as large as when moving from a non-care pathway to a paper-based care pathway environment. Consequently, computerised care pathway development teams will need to be fully engaged in service commissioning processes in their local health community. If this is not the case, the shifts in resources and the workforce changes that are required may well not materialise. The computerised care pathway could then fail because it is in effect too radical a change, even though it might be clinically and technically feasible. Figure 4.4 shows these pathway development choices schematically.

Conclusion

This case study of the stroke follow-up computerised care pathway pilot at Walsall demonstrates that pathways embedded in clinical computing systems allow:

- custom views of patient status and history tailored to the needs of specific professionals
- rapid and reliable communication between members of clinical teams and between computer systems
- automatic routing of referrals and task list reminders
- more flexible forms to both display and collect patient data at different stages of the pathway, which reduces duplication of data
- access to clinical records simultaneously from multiple locations at any time.

Computerised care pathways are qualitatively different from paper-based pathways because they address some significant limitations of the latter, and enable new ways of working which were too costly previously in a paper-based environment.

Important lessons have been learnt from this case study which need to be tested across other similar pilot projects to explore the extent of transferability of these issues within an NHS environment. If the lessons learnt at Walsall do prove generalisable across the wider NHS, then they will have important implications for anyone planning to develop computerised care pathways.

References

1 NHS Executive (1998) *Information for Health: an information strategy for the modern NHS 1998–2005.* Department of Health, London.
2 Department of Health (2002) *Delivering 21st Century IT Support for the NHS.* Department of Health, Leeds, http://www.doh.gov.uk/ipu/whatnew/deliveringit/index.htm.
3 Department of Health (1998) *A First Class Service: consultation document on quality in the new NHS.* HSC 1998/113. Department of Health, Leeds.
4 Rudd AG, Hoffman A, Irwin P and Lowe D on behalf of the Intercollegiate Stroke Working Party (2000) *National Sentinel Audit for Stroke: a tool for raising standards of care.* Royal College of Physicians, London, www.rcplondon.ac.uk.
5 Wade D and the Intercollegiate Working Party for Stroke (1999) *National Clinical Guidelines for Stroke.* Royal College of Physicians, London, www.rcplondon.ac.uk.
6 Department of Health (2001) *National Service Framework for Older People.* Department of Health, London.
7 Figures 4.1, 4.2 and 4.3 are copied with permission from: Walsall Middleware Partnership (2002) *Integrated Care Sub-Project Charter v1.*
8 Barthel scoring and over 3900 other medical algorithms are detailed at www.medal.org.
9 Sackett DL, Straus SE, Richardson WS, Rosenberg W and Haynes RB (2000) Asking answerable clinical questions. In: DL Sackett *et al.* (eds) *Evidence-based Medicine: how to practise and teach EBM* (2e). Churchill Livingstone, Edinburgh.

Appendix 4.1: Example screen shots

This appendix shows a few of the screens from the system developed by the Walsall stroke follow-up team so that readers who may not be familiar with the practicalities of electronic patient record systems and computerised care pathways can visualise concepts such as task lists and electronic forms.

While there are many computer systems in the market-place which provide similar features, in the UK health service at least, they are not commonplace.

In addition to the user screens, system administration screens not shown here would be used to set up and maintain the rules, staff roles, evidence links, computer interfaces, data sets, forms etc. required by each care pathway. Chapters 5 and 6 explore the possibility of more detailed information models for care pathways, which would help care pathway development teams to collate these additional details required for computerisation.

The screens are copyright and are provided courtesy of Orion Health (http://www.orionhealth.com).

Notes

1 Individual personal details have been blanked out.
2 Colour coding is used throughout the system (e.g. red text to indicate overdue tasks) – because this is not so clear in the black and white illustrations in this book, an electronic version of this appendix is on the CD.

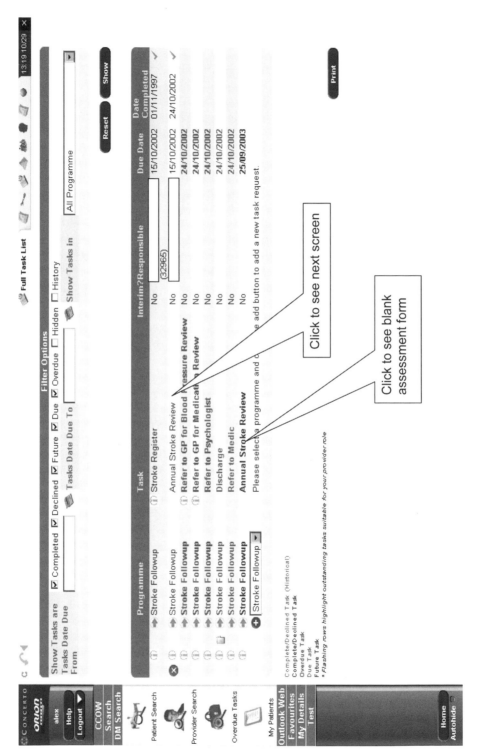

Figure 4A1.1 Full task list – full list of tasks for a patient; overdue, completed, due etc.

CONCERTO — ORION

alex
Help
Logout ▼
CCOW
Search
DM Search
Patient Search
Provider Search
Overdue Tasks
My Patients
Outlook Web
Favourites
My Details
Test

Home
Autohide

🗐 Full Task List   13:20 10/29

Programme/Task Name	Date Due	DateCompleted	Completion Status
Stroke Followup/Annual Stroke Review	15/10/2002	24/10/2002	Completed

History

	Date Due	DateCompleted	Completion Status
Diabetes	Oral Hypoglycaemic		
Hypertension	no		
		Cholesterol	Above 5 mmols

Lifestyle

	Date Due	DateCompleted	Completion Status
Smoker	yes	Smoking - no. per day	over 20
Diet	High Fat	Alcohol - Units/week	over 40

Medication Compliance

	Date Due	DateCompleted	Completion Status
Aspirin	Prescribed but non-co...		
Other Antiplatelet	Not Prescribed	Anticoagulant	Not Prescribed
Anti Hypertensive	Not Prescribed	Psychotropic	Prescribed but non-co...
Ace Inhibitor	Not Prescribed	Statin	Not Prescribed

Investigation

	Date Due	DateCompleted	Completion Status
BP Systolic	195 (mmHg)	Blood Glucose	27 (mmol/l)
BP Diastolic	95 (mmHg)		

HADS Score

	Date Due	DateCompleted	Completion Status
Anxiety	16	Depression	15

Crown ADL Index

	Date Due	DateCompleted	Completion Status
Bowels	2	Bladder	2
Toilet Use	1	Washing & Grooming	2
Dressing	1	Feeding	2
Communication	2	Transfers	1
Mobility	1	Stairs	0
Bathing	1	Awareness	0
Total Barthel (from Crown)	8.0	Total Crown	15.0

Print   Back

Figure 4A1.2 Completed task detail – shows a completed annual stroke review. (Entered from the completed annual stroke review shown on the full task list screen.)

Figure 4A1.3 Non-completed task – annual stroke review, shown as a future task on the full task list screen. Shown here as a blank form.

Figure 4A1.4 Non-completed task – annual stroke review, shown as a future task on the full task list screen. Shown immediately prior to pressing the complete button to complete the task.

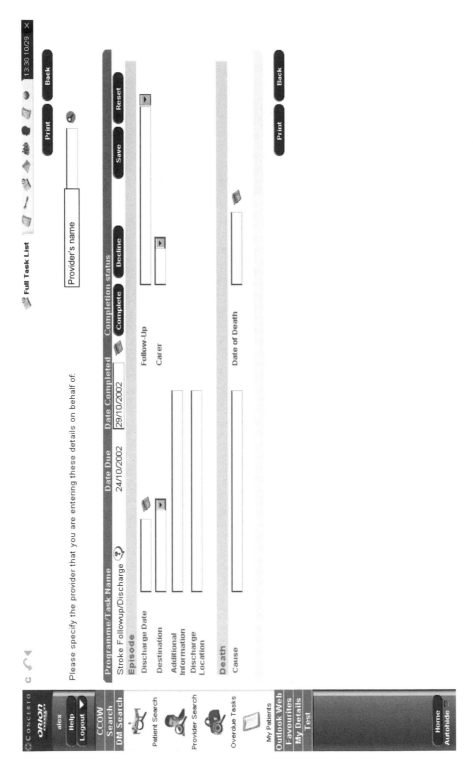

Figure 4A1.5 Another task completion screen – this one for a discharge task.

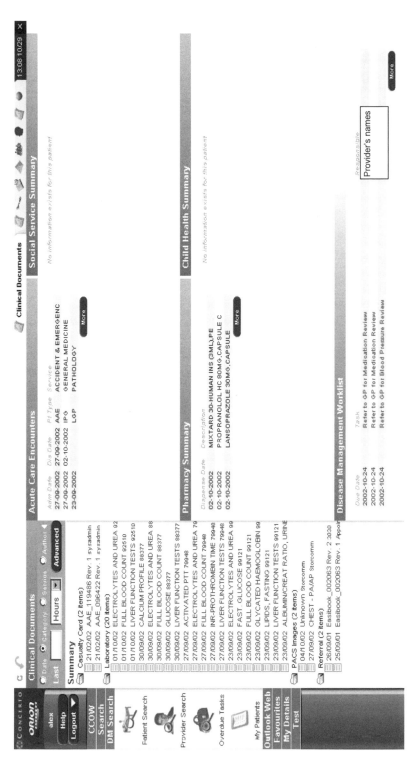

Figure 4A1.6 Dynamic patient summary screen – accessible by GPs. Note the view of overdue disease management tasks (bottom right). GPs can see that overdue tasks exist, but they cannot view details of the task or complete the task.

Part Two

Summary of main points

Chapters 5 and 6 explore issues which the editors and authors believe are essential to widespread adoption of computerised care pathways. The two chapters do, of necessity, introduce a number of concepts and approaches which may be less familiar to people with little knowledge of information technology. We have explained new concepts and ideas as they are used in non-technical language where possible, so we would obviously recommend all readers to tackle what we hope will be a useful and interesting part of the book. However, we are realists, so this brief summary of the main points will allow you to move on to the conclusions in Chapter 7 without losing the thread of the argument.

'Systems thinking' is essentially about building models as metaphors to help us to understand and shape the 'real world'. Care pathway developers are implicitly using the concept of a system model when they map the patient journey as part of their development process. Systems thinking is a very broad and rapidly developing field, which underpins many concepts and approaches which we increasingly take for granted. The following example concepts and terms are all derived from, or built upon, systems-based approaches – cyclic approaches to change management, feedback, process redesign, knowledge management, total quality management, governance, information technology, cybernetics, operations research, queue theory and learning organisations.

Paper-based pathways can work reasonably well using only locally agreed ways of modelling the patient journey. In systems terms, however, the resulting pathway documents are almost completely unsuited to implementation in clinical computer systems. Computerisation of care pathways presents new challenges, requiring more precise models of the clinical activities and choices which make up a care pathway. e-pathways must contain explicitly defined elements at a fine level of detail, including roles, tasks, sequence and timing, clinical rules, data definitions, messages, forms etc. As Chapter 4 showed, a computerised care pathway is not simply an automated version of its paper predecessor – clinical computer systems facilitate new ways of working, so robust approaches to process redesign at a whole community level are required.

Computerised care pathways require improved approaches based on proven systems modelling techniques. Systems models:

- always have explicitly defined parts and relationships
- are often standardised for common problems and areas of work
- can adapt to become as complex as they need to be to encompass all relevant aspects of the real world.

Chapter 5 explores aspects of systems theory and modelling which are relevant to change management, process redesign and care pathway modelling for development, implementation and maintenance of e-pathways at whole-community level.

Chapter 6 describes a possible definition and standard model of care pathways for use at national level when specifying clinical computer systems and exchanging/comparing care pathways.

A systems view of care pathways

Julian Todd

Key points

- The field of systems theory provides a number of concepts and techniques which are relevant to the development and implementation of care pathways.

- Several case studies show that it is both possible and beneficial for health communities to adapt systems and process-modelling approaches from commerce and industry.

- Computerised care pathways require detailed, structured definitions of their constituent elements, including roles, tasks, sequence and timing, clinical rules, data items, messages and forms. This level of detail in multiple care pathways is best managed at community level via special-purpose systems modelling software.

Introduction

The purpose of this chapter is to show how various systems-based approaches can be harnessed in the development and implementation of care pathways. A summary of some of the theory behind the approaches is provided and by way of several case studies the benefits are highlighted. Additional material on relevant systems theory and methods is provided on the CD accompanying this book, while many of the technical terms are defined in the glossary.

What is 'systems thinking' and what has it got to do with care pathways? From a systems perspective, care pathways are a challenging problem at any level – from individual pathway development, through whole organisation clinical effectiveness initiatives, to implementation of care processes in computer software.

Systems thinking as a discipline in its own right has, so far, had only a weak direct influence on care pathways and associated NHS organisational developments. In other areas of healthcare it is easy to find examples of complex systems approaches:

- research in human pathology, genetics and ultimately the nature of life itself as a complex, non-equilibrium system
- research and development of sophisticated medical equipment, new treatment approaches such as telemetric surgery and new drug therapies
- healthcare facilities design and build.

To answer the opening question, we need to go back to some basic principles and work forward to a richer view of how systems thinking can help in care pathway development and implementation.

Why model?

From a general viewpoint, systems thinking builds on the very old idea that it is helpful for people who are working together to solve a problem or design something to use *models*. The real world is complex and messy, so we take the essential aspects of reality relevant to a particular situation and create an idealisation. We can visualise and maybe simulate and predict what would happen in different circumstances. For complex problems, the model can provide common ground between different specialists' and world views – a framework for discussion, agreement and co-operative effort.

Care pathways are very good examples of this modelling approach – multidisciplinary teams working together to agree an ideal patient journey. In the real world of course, the ideal is rarely achieved, but at least there is a benchmark to compare and improve performance. The concept of such 'feedback loops' is itself a fundamental systems concept.

Systems thinking took the modelling concept and developed general principles, mathematical rigour where relevant and highly structured models suited to different situations. Post World War II, the systems community has developed a wide range of techniques and remains a rapidly developing field.[1-7]

A common theme running through most systems disciplines is the view that the whole is greater than the sum of the parts. This concept is variously labelled 'holistic', 'systemic', or 'whole systems'. Table 5.1, adapted from de Rosnay (1979),[8] contrasts the conventional scientific reductionist view or analytical approach with the systemic view, although it must be noted that in many practical situations these approaches are complementary.

Table 5.1 Comparison of reductionist/analytical approach to systemic approach

Reductionist approach	Systemic approach
Isolates, then concentrates on the elements.	Unifies and concentrates on the interaction between elements.
Studies the nature of interaction.	Studies the effects of interactions.
Emphasises the precision of details.	Emphasises global perception.
Modifies one variable at a time.	Modifies groups of variables simultaneously.
Remains independent of duration of time; the phenomena considered are reversible.	Integrates duration of time and irreversibility.
Validates facts by means of experimental proof within the body of a theory.	Validates facts through comparison of the behaviour of the model with reality.
Uses precise and detailed models that are less useful in actual operation.	Uses models that are insufficiently rigorous to be used as bases of knowledge but are useful in decision and action.
Has an efficient approach when interactions are linear and weak.	Has an efficient approach when interactions are non-linear and strong.
Leads to action programmed in detail.	Leads to action through objectives.
Possesses knowledge of details; goals poorly defined or absent.	Possesses knowledge of goals; fuzzy details.

Systems thinking is more like a way of looking at and interacting with the world in a methodical way than a conventional empirical scientific, analytical discipline. This makes it difficult to provide a universally accepted simple definition of 'system', but de Rosnay suggests:[8]

a system is a set of elements in dynamic interaction, organised for a goal.

Within healthcare we take for granted complex models based on systems thinking. For example:

- To understand and treat disease, clinicians use models of human pathology at various scales and levels of detail – from population-wide epidemiology, to whole body systems (e.g. nervous, endocrine etc.), to microbiological and cellular processes.
- The design and build of new hospitals requires, for example, models of modular construction systems, building engineering systems, project planning systems etc., which are the domain of technical specialists. These specialists interact with the client through architectural models of space and light, and the flow of people, materials, heat etc., which are embodied in 2D and 3D diagrams using symbols to represent real-world things. To participate in the building design process, we have to learn how to read the symbols.

Escalating costs, shortages of trained staff and rising expectations mean that many healthcare systems in the developed world are rethinking how they provide healthcare for their populations. Many healthcare systems are undergoing rationalisations, restructuring and redesign programmes. The NHS is no exception to this phenomenon. The NHS modernisation programme outlined in *The NHS Plan*[9] is a huge undertaking, far more complex and risky than building hospitals. Somehow, over the next decade or so, the NHS has to maintain services while changing the working lives of hundreds of thousands of people. Do we currently use models which are suited to the scale and complexity of this task? Are we organised properly to undertake this task? Do we have viable models of our organisations, how teams of people co-operate and how healthcare is delivered? Which aspects of systems thinking are relevant and how can they be applied to best effect?

A central theme of this book is that care pathways hold the key to these questions because they:

- require explicit thinking about effective teamwork during their development, implementation and application to individual patients
- embody an approach based on continuous improvement of care quality through reflection on variances or exceptions from ideal models of care

- focus on the 'patient journey' to create an explicit, process-based view of healthcare
- represent the point at which practical healthcare meets clinical computer systems, such as electronic patient record systems or protocol-based electronic referral and booking systems.

Thus, it would seem if we apply appropriate support to care pathways, we could obtain the significant leverage on healthcare systems needed to make the necessary changes to cope with 21st century demands and, in the UK context, to deliver on the modernisation agenda.

Care pathways from a systems perspective

In thinking about care pathways, there appear to be five limitations which have already been discussed in detail in Chapter 1. They are:

1 clinical evidence management at local, national and international levels
2 individual pathway development, implementation and maintenance
3 embedding pathways in clinical computer systems
4 how to use care pathways to support whole-community organisational change management
5 lack of clarity of concept and definitions for care pathways and related topics which are universally understood and accepted.

Previous chapters have explored issues 1–4 from a practitioner's point of view, while issue 5 is covered in Chapter 6. This chapter explores issues 1–4 from a systems perspective. The main systems problems in each of these four areas are summarised below:

Care pathway development
- achieving multidisciplinary, multi-agency teamworking
- incorporating evidence and best practice from elsewhere
- process mapping, analysis and redesign
- development of structured documentation
- personal and team development

Evidence management
- searches, cataloguing and citation
- evidence appraisal
- moderated evidence sources
- regular review and alerts

Organisation development/change management
- clinical authority for care pathway content and clinical governance frameworks for support and implementation

- whole-systems working and facilitation
- high-level processes and service redesign
- health community commissioning and workforce planning to manage the financial and human aspects of service redesign

Computerised care pathways
- definition of clinical data sets (e.g. lung cancer data set)
- design of on-screen forms and other user interface features (e.g. menu structures)
- definition of roles, tasks, sequencing and 'business rules' for 'clinical work-flow' at a fine level of detail, suitable for computerisation
- definition of messages to be exchanged between computer systems and people at key points in the pathway.

Outline requirement

The choice of systems approaches depends on the nature of what systems analysts call the 'system in focus'. If we are to cover adequately the issues outlined above, we will need a wide range of models and change techniques, including:

- individual team facilitation techniques
- research methods and knowledge management for evidence-based practice
- whole-organisation change management systems for quality assurance and maintenance of pathways, continuous quality improvement, workforce development, process redesign
- highly structured and detailed models for care pathways suitable for computerisation, including process steps, tasks, roles, data sets, decision charts, quantitative information such as cost, capacity, timing etc.

How can we tell whether a model is appropriate and effective? Models are tools for thinking about complex problems. Good models must:

- support consensus views of the world – all team members should understand the model, perhaps not in full or in exactly the same way, but well enough to be sure that when they apply the model to their real world, the desired changes are realised
- include metaphors for all *relevant* real-world features of the 'system in focus' – its components, processes and interrelationships. For example, to build a model of a car with a small child, you could use a couple of cereal packets to form the car body, a cardboard tube cut into four cylinders for the wheels and some bright paint. To train car mechanics,

you would need a far more sophisticated model so they could learn to diagnose, dismantle and reassemble the real thing. At the other extreme, car design and production is now so sophisticated that engineers specialise in one particular aspect of the whole machine, such as using complex computer models to improve engine efficiency.

Do models reflect reality?

Before discussing modelling and process redesign and their relevance to care pathways, it's worth highlighting two general points about models which are often left implicit:

1 When working with groups of people and models, what matters most for a positive outcome is consensus – there is no single reality which can be imposed from outside a group. Where human systems are concerned, all points of view or 'world views' should be regarded as equally valid (provided, of course, that they are internally consistent).
2 Complex, real-world systems – especially organisations – often behave in unexpected ways. Interventions may have little effect, or maybe even have the opposite effect to what was desired. If the people affected by a proposed change don't understand or support the proposal, then it probably won't happen.

The first point reflects the ongoing debate in systems thinking between 'hard systems' and 'soft systems' thinking and is closely related to the left and right columns in Table 5.1. Hard systems thinking (sometimes also called 'traditional' systems thinking) tends to believe that models truly reflect 'external reality'. This is a useful approach for many problems in science and engineering, but not for organisational change.

Soft systems methodology (SSM)[10] is an approach which has been developed as an alternative to hard (or traditional) systems analysis in the design and implementation of computer systems. It is one of a group of approaches which takes into account the human and social factors of organisations during systems design. When it was first developed, SSM focused on the structured, systemic modelling of human activity in organisations as perceived by the stakeholders, in order to design more successful information systems. As it has developed, the approach has acquired an increasing emphasis on cultural analysis, which has served to position it more specifically in the field of organisational change. SSM uses the term 'systemic' analysis, i.e. consensus-based modelling of 'whole systems', where the whole is greater than the sum of the parts. Contrast this with the reductionist approach of hard systems thinking, where an external expert 'analyst' interprets the statements of multiple stakeholders and designs a 'solution'. Case study 1 (*see* pp. 121–2) outlines how SSM has been used by one health community to support care pathway development.

The second point – that complex systems behave in unexpected ways – is the underlying rationale for a whole spectrum of approaches to change management and systems modelling. The issues of unexpected organisational behaviour are explored in more detail in, for example, Flood and Carson (1988)[11] and Forrester (1971).[12] Pratt *et al.* (1999)[13] provides an overview of systemic approaches.

In one sense, a patient journey through the health and social care system can be thought of as a chain of many queues – both physical and virtual – such as appointments to see particular healthcare professionals, undergo diagnostic tests and receive treatment. Care pathway development, especially computerised pathway development as shown in the previous chapter, involves redesigning the patient journey. As a result, the behaviour of the queues may change, indeed new queues may form around new services such as nurse-lead clinics. Queues of interest to care pathway development teams may be general-purpose – such as an appointment for a computed tomography (CT) scan – meaning that patients on that pathway are competing with all other patients requiring that service. Optimisation of such scarce resources therefore becomes a quality/performance issue for care pathway implementation.

Queue theory is a specific field of systems thinking, which is an interesting hybrid of soft and hard methods because it shows quantitatively how relatively simple rules frequently throw up unexpected behaviour in complex systems (e.g. transport network 'gridlock'). Queue theory has been applied to NHS capacity management in the form of the 'Big Wizard'.[14] Wilde (2002)[15] compares how various systems approaches, including queue theory, can be applied to an acute hospital CT scanning service. Although there is evidence of successful redesign of healthcare processes using static models, some health communities have taken the additional step of producing dynamic simulations, which help to identify true bottlenecks and realistic means of managing them.[16–18]

The theory of constraints (TOC)[19,20] – see Case study 2 – proposes that any complex, goal-oriented system can be thought of as a sequence of queues and that there will always be one queue which is the limiting factor or 'constraint' to maximum efficiency. TOC then defines a step-by-step approach to optimising the system and manage the constraint.

Given that the patient experience and, potentially, clinical outcomes are adversely affected by delays in treatment, it appears that care pathway development could benefit from what queue theory and TOC have discovered about how queues behave and how best to manage them.

This is likely to be more significant as the number of pathway and modernisation projects being undertaken at one time in a community increases.

A current difficulty for e-pathway development is that models from the soft systems end of the spectrum are often too vague to be directly implementable in IT systems. Hard systems models in contrast tend to be very detailed and precise, but this is different to 'true' in the sense of being owned and understood by all stakeholders. To computerise care pathways, we clearly need precise detail for the kind of reality we are trying to model. So, we need to find a middle ground – facilitation and change management approaches which are inclusive, open and creative – which have already been described in Chapter 3 – but which use models rich and precise enough to deal with the systems we are trying to change or implement.

Process redesign and e-pathways

Care pathway development teams usually 'map the patient journey', which may include drawing a process map. The term or methodology 'business process re-engineering' (BPR) has sometimes been applied to this aspect of care pathways.[21] BPR is a relatively recent change management approach which originated in large corporations in the USA.[22,23] A range of definitions exist, but in essence BPR involves radical redesign, focusing on efficiency and the value provided to the customer in goods and services.

Care pathway development does not appear to be a BPR programme in the sense used by the original authors because the former has more in common with gradual quality improvement approaches. BPR proponents such as Hammer and Stanton (1995)[24] stress the radical nature of BPR.

When discussing how to map the patient journey in a form suitable for computerisation, the term 'process redesign' is therefore preferred in this book rather than 'BPR' because the latter is misleading in this context, due to its emphasis on radical, rapid change. See Darnton and Darnton (1997)[25] for a detailed survey of the field.

However, to implement care pathways in computer software we do require a precise framework for modelling and redesigning business processes within healthcare. Some of the thinking and techniques developed by the BPR community may therefore have something to offer. Compare the following quote from a key BPR author, with the requirement that care pathways are 'patient-focused':[26]

[Business process] re-engineering entails as great a shift in the culture of an organisation as in its structural configuration. Re-engineering demands that employees deeply believe they work for their customers, not for their bosses.

Process redesign is still more of an art than a science. However, equally clearly there are ways of managing a redesign project and specific modelling techniques which yield a greater chance of success. Mayer *et al.* (1999)[27] summarise experience of case studies as showing these common reasons for BPR projects failures, which could alternatively be called risk factors:

- multiple, unco-ordinated activities
- lack of commitment to establishing an in-house (organic) capability
- insufficient or inadequate methodology, methods, tools
- attempts to outsource key decision making
- failure to concurrently address business, information system and organisational change together with process change
- inability to leverage information technologies and realign information systems quickly enough to make a smooth transition
- inability to align process intent with organisational vision and goals, structure and job performer management
- lack of top-level commitment and understanding.

These risk factors can also provide a useful benchmark and check-list for the process redesign and change management aspects of care pathway development at organisation/community and possibly also national level.

There is plenty of best practice specific to healthcare process redesign, such as the NHS Modernisation Agency publications.[28] However, the process modelling techniques promoted so far by the NHS modernisation programme and others are not detailed or precise enough for computerisation of care pathways. There has also been relatively little work to date on the relationship between clinical computer systems and their potential for facilitating new working practices and more efficient processes as part of care pathway development and implementation.

Modelling and change at whole-organisation level

Although care pathway development can occur in isolated teams, it is far more effective to work within a whole organisation (or preferably a whole health community) context. As Lathrop *et al.* described the situation in 1988:[29]

> To be meaningful and sustainable, operations improvement must be approached at a higher level, using the same long-term, analytical, creative process employed in strategic planning.

The details differ, but all change management approaches are based on an explicit methodology and a cyclic approach to change. For example, Figure 5.1 shows the overall process recommended by the Commission for Health Improvement (CHI) to support clinical audit.[30]

One of the problems with methodologies is that authors tend to promote them as universal, whereas in practice they are just like models. None of them are *correct*; they are merely more or less useful in particular situations.[31] Even if a methodology is appropriate to the nature of the problem, it must still be owned and understood by the participants in order to be effective – it cannot be followed blindly as a set of rules.

Many systems models of organisations, including the organisational boundaries and hierarchies which we encounter on a daily basis, are focused on stability and control – *homeostasis* to use an organic systems analogy. However, 'patient journeys' regularly cross departmental and agency boundaries. These boundaries are there partly to provide a stable

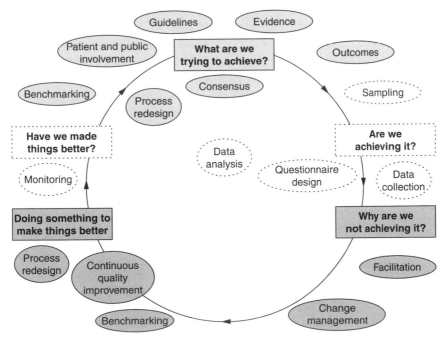

Figure 5.1 Cyclical change management as applied to clinical audit.[30]

organisational framework. Analysing and redesigning care pathways and implementing clinical computer systems necessarily challenge the *status quo* and potentially destabilise organisations.

For change management, we need models of *metamorphosis* – ordered change. Kurt Lewin, who laid the foundation for the organisational development (OD) movement, described a three-phase model of change which involved the unfreezing, moving and refreezing of configurations.[32] Softened plastic rather than flowing liquid might be a more helpful image, however – liquid tends to flow in unpredictable ways unless its movement is limited by rigid external constraints.

Perhaps through conscious choice to avoid such risks of unpredictability, clinical governance initiatives, including care pathway development, have tended towards gradual change approaches derived from management science such as total quality management (TQM) and theory of constraints. See Case study 2 below for an example of the use of the TOC in redesigning services.

The gradualist approach has a downside, however, because it has contributed to a trend toward devolution of effort and co-ordination to small speciality teams. Sufficient resources and co-ordination have often not been available at local organisational or whole-community level and, as argued later in Chapter 7, at national level. Within the context of care pathways there has been a resulting tendency towards inefficiency, patchy progress and difficulties in achieving lasting change.

The rest of this chapter contains a number of examples of different systems approaches which have been used by healthcare organisations/communities for process redesign and care pathway development. Firstly there are four short case studies which illustrate the way systems thinking has achieved quality improvements in healthcare. The final section describes in more detail a particular approach taken by one acute NHS trust to use systems modelling software to support both a structured model for its computerised care pathway development and its whole-community change programmes.

Case study examples

This section of the chapter includes four illustrative case studies taken from various projects around the UK. The first case study shows the use of soft systems methodology to support a stroke pathway development team. The second case study shows how a change technique called theory of constraints can be used in process redesign to support improved patient journeys. The third case study shows how clinical guidelines presented in a flow-chart format and made available at the point of care can assist clinical staff in their decision making. This use of decision support in the form of flow diagrams is commonly found in care pathway design. The fourth case study shows how process mapping – again using flow-chart conventions – can be utilised on a large scale, across agencies. In themselves, these four case studies are not complete and comprehensive care pathways. They do, however, illustrate how systems aproaches can be utilised for some of the key elements of pathways.

The main conclusions which can be drawn from these case studies include:

- High-level ownership and clinical leadership, coupled with central facilitation, is critical.
- Clinical teams can think in process terms and use complex symbolic diagrams, provided the conventions used are made relevant and clear.
- Methodologies developed for industry/commerce can work in healthcare if adapted sensitively.
- Whole systems approaches are commonly used to build consensus in multi-professional and multi-agency teams.
- Significant operational benefits can be obtained through process redesign, without necessarily pouring in extra resources.

Case study 1 Using soft systems methodology in the development of a stroke care pathway

Sarah Caldicott, Integrated Care Pathway Co-ordinator, Hereford Acute Hospitals

Sandi Kirkham, Principal Lecturer, School of Computing, University of Central England in Birmingham

Helen Sudlow, Clinical Governance Co-ordinator, Herefordshire Primary Care Trust

A care pathway for stroke care has recently been identified as a priority pathway project in Herefordshire. However, the needs of stroke patients are diverse; no two patients are the same. Facilitating the individual needs of a patient who has had a stroke, and ensuring all stakeholder aims are achieved, is a challenge for the healthcare service, and for a care pathway.

The stroke pathway in Herefordshire is being developed using Checkland's soft systems methodology. SSM has been applied to the development of the stroke care pathway in Hereford for three reasons:

- The delivery of stroke care is complex and multidisciplinary, involving a wide range of medical expertise and other agencies such as social services and carer associations. An approach was required which would enable as many stakeholders as possible to become involved in the development of the pathway and encourage a strong sense of commitment and co-operation.
- An egalitarian approach was required which would help to break down some of the hierarchical barriers which might exist within the stakeholder group.
- SSM enables the information systems requirements of activity models to be specified, therefore providing a tool for the development of an electronic pathway to support the stroke care pathway. This feature could also help to break down some of the barriers and misconceptions about the use of electronic care systems within the development team.

The starting point for the pathway development was an extensive stakeholder analysis to ensure that everyone involved in stroke care was involved (*see* Figure 5.2). It is worth noting the position of the patient at the centre of the stakeholder analysis. The views of stroke patients were represented by both patients themselves, and carer group representatives.

The next step was to encourage commitment from all these stakeholders, and individual interviews. Multidisciplinary workshops were conducted to provide information about SSM and gain individual views of stroke care. Each view was modelled and presented to the stakeholder for feedback and possible modification. A series of workshops were held involving as many stakeholders as possible, during which all the models were debated. The outcome of this process was the development of an agreed conceptual model illustrating the 'ideal' patient journey for stroke care (*see* Figure 5.3).

The concept of a care pathway suggests a more linear entity than is represented by the conceptual model. Its value was found to be the way it identified the key activities involved in stroke care and their interrelationships, particularly information flows. For example, activity 4a shows an input coming from activity 4, indicating that the *information* produced by doing activity 4 is required by activity 4a. The SSM conceptual map is therefore a richer picture of the patient journey than the 'traditional' process map. The fact that the final conceptual model is a consensus made up of many individual views strengthens the degree of ownership and commitment gained from using SSM.

The agreed model represents a high-level view of the patient journey. Each activity within this model is being developed, through the same process, into a further set of activities for each area. An example of an activity chart for activity 4a is shown in Figure 5.4. Using all the models, a check-list of care activities will be derived along with a variance data sheet to provide information about what is actually happening to stroke patients. These four elements (i.e. the agreed model, models of each activity, the activity check-lists and variance sheets) will be used as a clinical pilot, and it is hoped that this will take the project into clinical use.

In the short term, an interim paper-based care pathway will be developed until the electronic systems are developed to support a fully electronic, patient-centred, cross-agency pathway. The longer-term aim is to link clinical activity and evidence (from, for example, guidelines, protocols and procedures) electronically.

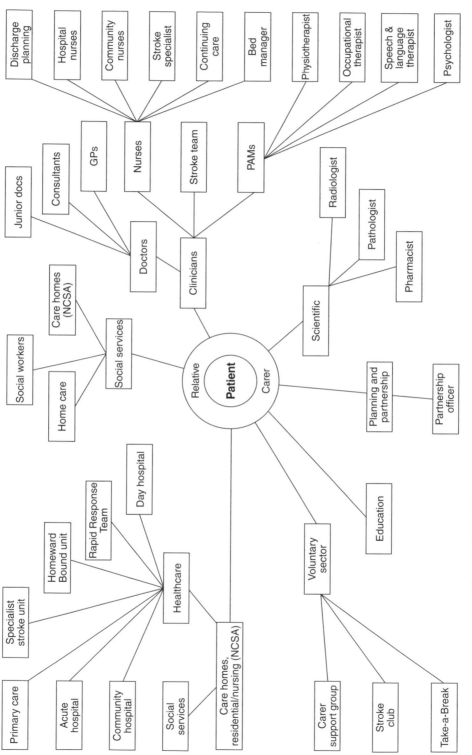

Figure 5.2 Hereford stroke care pathway stakeholder analysis.

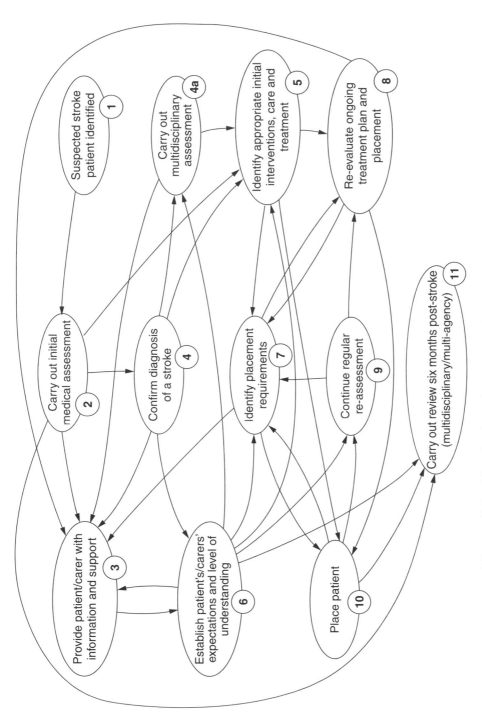

Figure 5.3 Hereford stroke care pathway conceptual model.

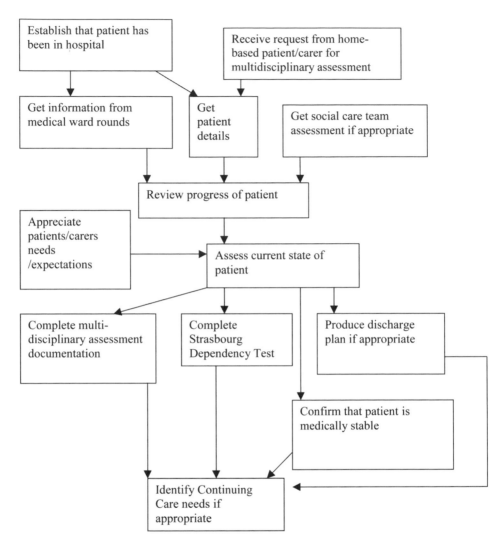

Figure 5.4 Hereford stroke care pathway – SSM activity chart 4a: 'Carry out multidisciplinary assessment'.

Case study 2 Applying the theory of constraints in Oxfordshire

Sarah Ives and Sally Reid, Redesign & Development Leads, Oxfordshire Patient Access Improvement Team (Host organisation – Oxford Radcliffe Hospitals Trust)

Significant operational improvements have been achieved by adapting a change management approach called theory of constraints to the NHS at Oxford Radcliffe Hospitals Trust. The theory of constraint was devised by Eliyahu Goldratt in the late 1970s and has been used extensively in industry both in the UK and in the USA. It is a management approach that focuses on whole systems, which aims to improve throughput without making the system work harder.

The TOC can be thought of as a refinement of the basic Plan-Do-Study-Act (PDSA) change cycle (Deming, 1989*). More information can be found on the accompanying CD, but the key point is that Goldratt's theory proposes that *all* systems have a constraint which limits throughput. The constraint may not be obvious. Sarah and Sally's adaptation of the TOC to healthcare includes whole systems workshops and process mapping to help identify the constraint. Once it has been identified, the TOC focuses on supporting the constraint to get the most out of it before any additional resources are put in.

At Horton General Hospital, there were significant problems with A&E trolley waits over 12 hours and high numbers of elective cancellations. From May to December 2001 a multidisciplinary/multi-agency team used the TOC approach, to cut excessive trolley waits per month from 28 down to one and reduce cancellations by over one half.

The Horton team identified 'nursed beds' as the constraint, analysed how it was being (mis)used and then systematically reduced the unnecessary pressures. In their case, this involved changes such as improved medical/surgical assessment, more efficient diagnostics and increased focus on discharge. The work highlighted the need to pull the patients through the system and has shifted the responsibility of managing capacity from individual departments to the whole health system.

Although the redesigned service was not explicitly implemented as a care pathway, the TOC approach and patient-centred view is clearly of interest as a care pathway development technique.

*Deming WE (1989) *Out of the Crisis*. MIT Press, Cambridge, MA.

Case study 3 FlowForma clinical guidelines website

Chris Taylor, Clinical Director (rtd.) A&E, Queen Mary's Hospital, Sidcup

The organisation identified through an audit study that adherence to clinical guidelines for asthma treatment was poor. The main reason was that the existing guidelines were not available in a suitable form when and where they were needed in the clinical area.

The existing guideline by the British Thoracic Society, which was already in quasi-flow-chart format, was converted into a 'pro forma in flow-chart form' – or 'FlowForma'. This removed the need to 'read' the guideline – the new simplified format was sufficient to guide staff through the process.

The approach was rapidly extended to other conditions with similar results. Variations in treatment were reduced, take-up rate was improved, feedback from nurses, junior medical staff and new members of staff was supportive of the direct, simple approach.

Various staff initiated FlowForma charts in response to need and Chris Taylor oversaw the evidence research and standardised the 'style' of the flow charts. Because the charts were developed and used locally, rapid development was possible to respond to queries and resolve disagreements about best practice.

The FlowForma charts are now available online at www.flow forma.org/ funded directly by Chris Taylor. The approach and the website have been so successful that he received a BMA award for 'consultants leading change'.

Case study 4 Process mapping in West Sussex Primary Care

Lisa Day, Process Mapping Co-ordinator, West Sussex Shared Services Consortium

The West Sussex GP Mapping Project is one of several similar undertakings in the area since 1998.

The objectives of the project were to produce patient-centred process maps of general practice, improve primary care teamworking and identify the main requirements for an integrated information support system. Eight representative practices were selected and each practice identified a multi-professional team, led by a 'process worker'. With the support of the central facilitation team, the process workers received training in the process modelling approach and facilitation techniques. Backfill funding was made available to help release staff time from clinical duties.

Where necessary, 'whole systems' workshops were run in addition to detailed process mapping to ensure that core processes and broader issues were properly identified, and that senior management and clinical buy-in to the project were in place. Some processes were mapped once and shared among all practices, while others were mapped by all practices and then compared in larger workshops to yield a consensus view.

All the process-mapping projects have adopted a hybrid modelling approach based on standard flow-chart diagrams plus annotations showing clinical information requirements/products at key stages of the process. Although most process maps are very detailed and self-contained, some work has been done in linking them and making them more specific to a patient condition to generate, e.g. a diabetes care pathway. Examples are shown in Figures 5.5 and 5.6. Further details of the project, including more example process maps, can be found on the accompanying CD.

Many benefits have been identified and the approach has been so successful that it has been adopted by all health/social care agencies in the area. The main benefits include:

- improved care processes through integration and sharing of information
- improved teamworking and inter-professional knowledge
- sense of ownership of redesigned ways of working
- basis for clinical governance and care pathway development
- improved strategic decisions on ICT, including gap analysis and baseline business case and improved communications with system suppliers.

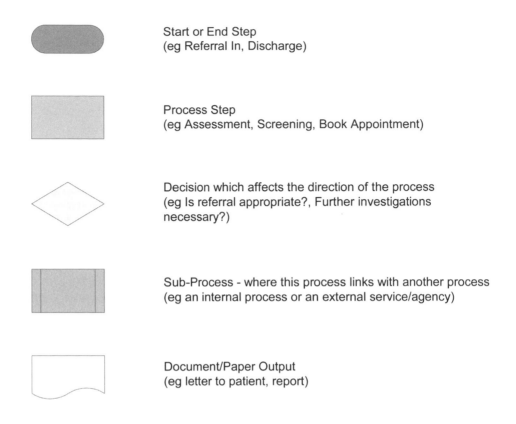

Start or End Step
(eg Referral In, Discharge)

Process Step
(eg Assessment, Screening, Book Appointment)

Decision which affects the direction of the process
(eg Is referral appropriate?, Further investigations
necessary?)

Sub-Process - where this process links with another process
(eg an internal process or an external service/agency)

Document/Paper Output
(eg letter to patient, report)

Red text = Information which is generated or changed by the process

Blue text = Information which is used by the process, but generated elsewhere

NOTE: To differentiate between blue text and red text in the black and white illustrations in this book, a ✳ symbol has been added to Figure 5.6 next to the blue text

Figure 5.5 Key to GP flow charts.

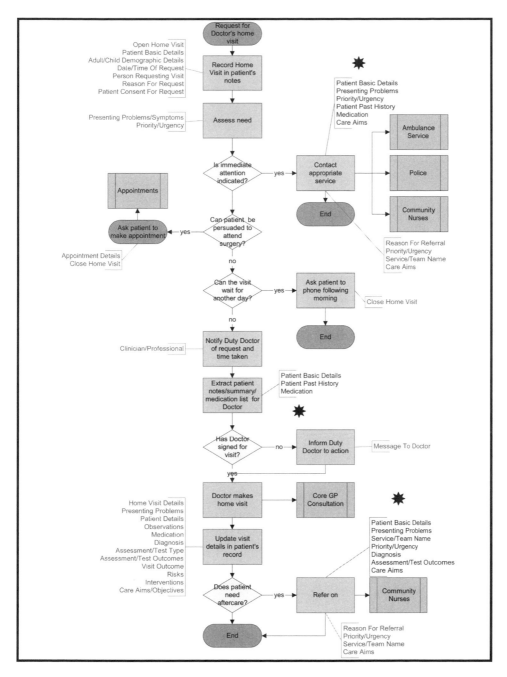

Figure 5.6 Example of GP flow chart – home visit.

Dudley change programme

The rest of this chapter builds on the analysis in the first part of the chapter and the lessons which can be learnt from the case studies. This section describes the approach taken in the Dudley healthcare community where a systems approach is being designed to help develop and implement computerised care pathways. The work involves both detailed process models and care pathway specifications within a whole-community change programme framework.

Because readers may wish to experiment with the modelling approach used in this example, a trial version of the software and example models can be found on the CD. Note that the change programme and modelling tool kit is at the very early stages of a development programme which is expected to last several years – these models are provided only to illustrate how the tool is used and do not represent real processes or care pathways.

Background

The modelling work in Dudley is happening in the context of a long-term plan for £160m investment in acute services, funded by a large Public Finance Initiative (PFI) scheme, which will in turn free up recurring funding for development of primary care. Dudley is a mainly urban community in the West Midlands area of England.

A multi-agency change programme, including primary, acute and social care representatives, was created to manage the new ways of working and revised working relationships associated with the design and configuration of the new acute facilities which are due to be completed in 2004/05. An overall board of senior stakeholder representatives plus several change teams were established, supported by a central facilitation team, and covering:

- high-level acute clinical services review
- workforce development
- a framework for service user consultation and involvement
- a highly detailed model of care pathways to support their development in a form suitable for computerised implementation
- electronic patient record systems implementation, including a care pathway module
- primary care change management
- building construction and co-ordination of service moves
- facilities management for the PFI scheme.

To date, over ten Clinical Services Review teams have been established. Some teams cover changes in working practices for specific professions or patient groups (e.g. new general nursing care model, new maternity care model). Most, however, are concerned to a greater or lesser degree with process redesign (e.g. emergency admissions, discharge co-ordination). The service review teams are working with other 'whole systems' change programme areas such as cancer services. All teams also work within a common framework, including workforce development, financial/contractual issues, service user consultation etc.

Each of these teams may identify specific care pathways and protocols which would aid implementation of the new ways of working. The 'top-down' approach to process redesign is based on the three main types of patient interaction with acute services – emergency, elective and out-patients. The approach will create overall templates, which can be developed at finer levels of detail as required by care pathway teams. These care pathway teams are made up of clinical staff supported by other professionals to ensure, for example, that the potential of the EPR system is maximised.

The change programme will last several years – to at least 2005/06 – and will establish a network of links with other major projects such as the implementation of the National Service Frameworks,[33,34] Booked Admissions,[35] and local implementation strategy for *Information for Health*.[36] Existing care pathway teams working 'bottom-up' designing individual care pathways will be supported to incorporate their work into the framework and computerise appropriate parts of their paper-based pathways.

The scale of the change programme is significant, involving many teams, significant large- and small-scale process redesign, and ultimately, it is hoped, many electronic care pathways. Given the scale of the undertaking it was felt that conventional means of co-ordination and communication would not be sufficiently structured, efficient or rapid. Therefore two key software tools were implemented:

- *Systems Architect*™ systems modelling software from Popkin Software and Systems Ltd[37]
- a community-wide intranet, accessible to both health service and borough council staff as the core of a communications framework.

The systems modelling software and associated care pathway model is explored in more detail below. Figure 5.7 shows a schematic of the Dudley communications framework. A recurring theme in change management projects, especially care pathway development, is the difficulty of assembling multi-agency and multidisciplinary teams for face-to-face meetings. Experience from other fields shows that software generally labelled 'computer supported cooperative work' can reduce the need for face-to-face meetings and improve overall communications by creating a 'virtual community' (*see* Chapter 3, Appendix 3.2) – at the time of writing the Dudley community is implementing a system called 'snitz' (www.snitz.com). This element of the communications framework is therefore shown in a dotted box in Figure 5.7.

The benefits of using systems modelling software

The main innovation in Dudley is the use of the *Systems Architect* modelling software. To understand the benefits of systems modelling software we first need to critically examine the relatively simple diagramming methods and tools used hitherto by most care pathway and NHS modernisation teams. Historic approaches to care pathway development have produced word-processed documents, which may or may not include diagrams of the 'patient journey'. In the context of implementation of care pathways in clinical computer systems, Table 5.2 shows, in the left column, a critique of 'traditional' approaches and in the right-hand column, the comparative benefits of systems modelling software for developing process maps and redesigning services as part of e-pathway development.

The two critical issues are that:

1 the detail and precision within the care pathway definition has to be maintained at a higher level to support computerisation of pathways
2 the care pathway definition must be maintained independently from the systems in which it is implemented because these will change over time and are always likely to require different approaches (including paper forms) in different agencies and circumstances.

Another way of looking at systems modelling software is to compare it directly with common alternatives such as word processors (e.g. *Microsoft Word*^{TM}), or more specialised drawing software (e.g. *Microsoft Visio*^{TM}). Table 5.3 compares *Systems Architect* with these other tools.

Because *Systems Architect* is built on a database, it has additional general benefits:

• It can grow to include all the interrelated detail of a large-scale change programme and multiple care pathways.
• It supports reuse of standard elements in many different care pathways and contexts, ranging from specific diagnostic tests (e.g. full blood count), through elementary processes (e.g. admit patient), to large-scale templates of care (e.g. elective surgery).
• Many people can access and update it simultaneously.

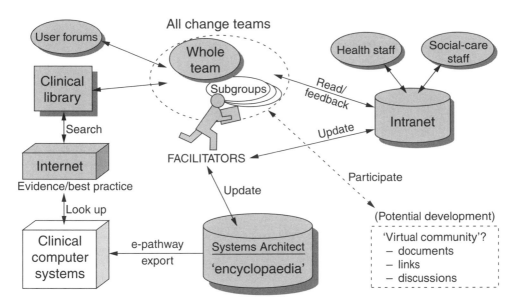

Figure 5.7 Dudley change programme – communications framework.

- Parts of it can be 'locked' and made read-only – to protect reference data such as pathology test definitions, for example, or to allow specific teams to 'book out' and 'book in' their own draft designs.
- Reports can be produced on particular parts of the database, either as structured text or in web format for direct publication on the community-wide intranet, which is helpful for creating a rapid feed-back loop to change-team members and the wider staff community.
- High-level and low-level views can be linked to help overcome the common problem with complex models of being 'unable to see the wood for the trees'.

What does systems modelling software do?

The fundamental difference between *Systems Architect* and the relatively simple diagramming methods and tools used by many care pathway teams and change programmes is that it uses 'symbolic modelling'. The outline of systems thinking earlier in this chapter established the role of models as metaphors for the real-world. We use diagrams to represent real-world things and relationships between them. In symbolic modelling software, all symbols have a defined meaning and there is a two-way relationship between symbols and the definitions of the things they represent. All diagrams, symbols, definitions and their interrelationships are stored in the encyclopaedia.

Table 5.2 Benefits of systems modelling software

Issue/problem of traditional approach	Feature/benefit of systems modelling
Diagrams are merely pictures and contain no information about the content and relationships between the things in the model, except in the 'eye of the beholder'. There is no relationship between diagrams and the text in the care pathway documentation.	Definitions of the things in the model, and their interrelationships are held in a database or 'encyclopaedia'. Diagrams become both views into, and part of, the database, not merely pictures.
For large projects, it is virtually impossible to track where things in the model are used and to ensure that all teams are using the same definitions.	The definitions in the database can be reused in different contexts. If a definition is changed, the changes are automatically reflected everywhere it is used. The database can report on where a definition is used.
Diagrams are often constructed from a few simple elements – lines, arrows, boxes. The meaning of these symbols *may* be clear to individual team members, but cannot be reliably interpreted by other people. Often, insufficient symbols are used to represent the richness of what is being modelled, so symbols become ambiguous. For example, boxes might be used on the same diagram to represent any of: a process, a decision, a goal or the status of a patient.	The modelling tool kit supports many standard systems models, appropriate to different design and change management problems. These standard models have explicit definitions of the types of things and relationships which they represent, which improves clarity of communications between care pathway teams and between clinical and IT staff.
Lack of diagramming standards hampers attempts to validate pathway development approach and content.	The quality of the models can be validated against the standards.
At a whole-organisation level, several modelling approaches will be required for different purposes.	Selected types of standard model can be combined to support specific change methodologies.
Care pathways are a unique systems/process modelling problem.	The standard definitions can be extended and adapted to include features required by a particular problem. Thus in Dudley, *Systems Architect* has been modified to include a highly structured definition of care pathways.

Table 5.3   Feature comparison of software tools for process modelling

	Pictures	Links between graphic objects	Definitions of objects	Reuse of definitions via 'encyclopaedia'	Support for modelling standards	Multi-user
Word	✓	Partial	✗	✗	✗	✗
Visio	✓	✓	Partial	✗	Partial	✗
Systems Architect	✓	✓	✓	✓	✓	✓

In Figure 5.8, these principles are shown schematically through the example of 'Radiology' as a department or 'organisational unit', with a definition (name, description etc.), which is represented using different symbols on different types of diagram. In Figure 5.8, 'Diagram 1' is an organisation chart, where departments are shown as boxes and the lines joining boxes represent management authority/responsibility. 'Diagram 2' is a process chart, where departments may be shown as 'swim-lanes' containing processes, so that it is clear which departments carry out which processes in the overall picture. If the underlying definition of Radiology changed, all symbols linked to the definition would 'see' the change. Reports could be generated from the encyclopaedia showing, for example, which diagrams used the Radiology organisational unit and which processes occurred within Radiology.

Outline of Dudley model structure

A number of models have been developed in the Dudley *Systems Architect* encyclopaedia which reflect the scope of the clinical services review and care pathway development programme. The main model types include:

- organisation (hierarchy)
- functional hierarchy/functional interdependence
- high-level maps of overall processes which can be both overall templates for e.g. elective surgery, or the whole of a specific care pathway reflecting the patient journey (e.g. total hip replacement)
- low-level, detailed process charts reflecting specific protocols, e.g. administration of thrombolysis for chest pain cases or stabilisation of

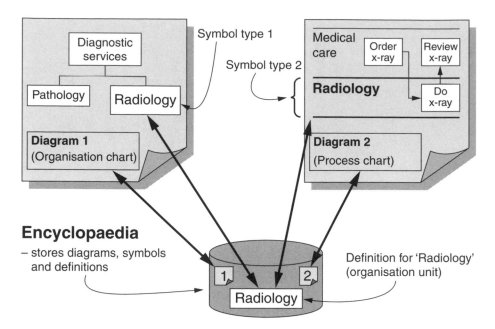

Figure 5.8 Essentials of symbolic modelling.

glucose levels for a patient with diabetic ketoacidosis (see example below)
* detailed definitions of each part of a care pathway and other model elements required by the change programme.

A structured definition of a care pathway has been developed which is designed to address the following issues:

* ongoing management of a growing number of pathways, capable of supporting several hundred individual pathways if required eventually
* the need to implement some stages of care pathways in computer software – principally the acute Electronic Patient Record (EPR) system, but potentially also primary care EPR systems and electronic booking systems, all of which require a highly structured, detailed and unambiguous representation of processes, tasks, roles, data sets, forms, messages etc.
* consistent use of standard elements of pathways such as a catalogue of investigative tests
* a standard framework for quality assurance of the pathway development process and products
* a mechanism for embedding into the EPR, hyperlinks to the pathway evidence base to provide basic decision support.

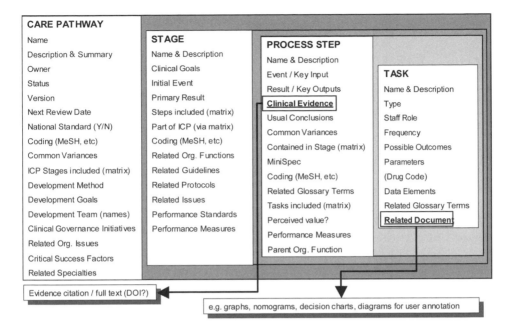

Figure 5.9 Care pathway definition comprising of stages, process steps and tasks.

Figure 5.9 shows a schematic of the whole care pathway model, where the pathway contains one or more stages, which contain one or more process steps, which contain one or more tasks. Stages and process steps can also be shown on related process maps and process charts respectively (see below). In *Systems Architect* we can move in both directions between diagrams and definitions. *Systems Architect* also allows hyperlinks to documents and websites to be embedded in the definition, so that if a particular step or task includes a clinical guideline, decision chart etc., a single click of a mouse will call up the document or website. This referencing mechanism can also support the Digital Object Identifier standard described in Chapter 2.

The care pathway model includes:

- information about the pathway itself ('meta-data') to aid version control and cataloguing. To reinforce the links between pathways and their evidence base, cataloguing data in the model is coded using one or more international standards such as Medical Subject Headings (MeSH)[38] or Cumulative Index to Nursing and Allied Health Literature (CINAHL)[39]
- additional meta-data to hold information required by the care pathway quality assurance process

- cross-references to other entities within the Dudley model, such as organisational units, organisational goals or national targets etc., for example the target for administration of thrombolysis within the Coronary Heart Disease National Service Framework
- detailed definitions of process steps, individual tasks, roles, data sets for clinical documentation and messages, common variances etc.
- Citations and hyperlinks to clinical evidence.

A care pathway defined in this highly structured way can be exported from the encyclopaedia and implemented either on paper (e.g. for a pilot) or in a clinical computer system. Work is ongoing in Dudley with the EPR supplier to export the care pathway definition in a format which can be directly imported into the EPR software. If this can be achieved it will save significant clinical and IT staff time.

As noted above, for care pathway process modelling and redesign, the Dudley model includes two interrelated types of diagram – high-level process maps and lower level process charts. Using two types of diagram overcomes one of the difficulties with the conventional approach to process mapping – how to get all the relevant detail onto the page.

Figure 5.10 shows schematically how high-level processes are decomposed into finer detail using these two types of diagram. The high-level process map contains several stages – shown as rounded rectangles.

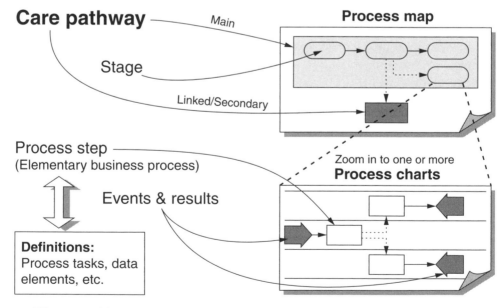

Figure 5.10 Mapping the patient journey using process maps and process charts.

Examples of stages would be 'GP consultation', 'GP to consultant referral', 'patient discharge' etc. Stages are joined by either 'mandatory sequence' lines – shown as solid arrows, or 'optional sequence' lines – the dotted arrows. A stage can have many incoming and outgoing lines to represent optional flow sequences. When modelling care pathways, we group several stages together into a larger rectangular container which represents the whole pathway. On the same diagram we can also show links to other whole pathways – indicated in Figure 5.10 by the small rectangle below the main care pathway rectangle. For example, the chest pain and myocardial infarction care pathway described in Chapter 2 is in two parts, reflecting the symptom stage of chest pain and the diagnosis stage when a myocardial infarction is confirmed. This can link directly to an angina whole care pathway.

Process maps are used to develop and show the 'whole picture', but on their own they cannot show sufficient detail. For this, the Dudley model uses process charts. We can literally 'zoom in' to the detail of each stage using one or more process charts, depending on the complexity of the stage. The rule of thumb is how much detail can be shown legibly on one sheet of paper, although *Systems Architect* can 'tile' large single diagrams onto multiple pages if required.

Process charts use a new set of symbols, only some of which are shown in Figure 5.10 for clarity. The main symbol is an 'elementary business process', shown as a rectangle, which is the symbol for a process step in the care pathway model shown in Figure 5.9 above. The Dudley model extends the standard definition of an elementary business process to include elements relevant to care pathways, so that from the process step on the process chart it is possible to build up the detail required to implement the care pathway in a clinical computer system.

The process chart also emphasises that stages are triggered by *events* (normally only one or two) and end with one or more *results*. Both are shown by inward-pointing arrows to highlight the start and end of the stage. The main purpose of including events and results in the model is to focus attention on the transition between stages, which often occurs between agencies, departments and professions. When care pathway and other process redesign teams talk of 'streamlining' or 'smoothing' the patient flow, what they mean in practice includes ensuring that:

- the decisions required are clear
- required conditions/patient status are met (these are normally 'clinical goals')
- transfer of responsibility is clear
- all the information required 'downstream' is available

- transfer of the patient, and any equipment and information required, is as efficient and quick as possible.

The importance of looking at a care pathway as a sequence of queues was discussed earlier in this chapter. Events on process charts are often the point at which a patient reaches the front of the queue. This approach to mapping the patient journey can therefore support whole systems redesign.

Although the care pathway model may appear complex at first sight, it contains no elements which are not already handled by 'traditional' best practice pathway development methods. The additional material is what is needed to efficiently manage the precision and structure required for the implementation of multiple care pathways in clinical computer systems. If required, any care pathway developed and maintained in the model can still be published in paper form for piloting and approval. Moreover, the modelling approach encourages progressive development of the detail and the reuse of standard stages, steps and tasks.

For a change programme on the scale outlined above, it was felt that the use of symbolic modelling software and a structured care pathway model was an essential element of a successful strategic approach to large-scale, long-term organisational change and the e-pathway development and implementation programme.

Appendices 5.1 and 5.2 show how the model can be applied in practice. The whole of a diabetic ketoacidosis (DKA) care pathway provided by Worcester is shown as a document in Appendix 5.1. Appendix 5.2 then shows the whole DKA pathway as a process map. One stage is then shown as a process chart, and within this parts of the definitions of a process step and a task are shown. This treatment of the DKA pathway can be compared with the same pathway analysed using the proposed national Care Pathway Conceptual Structure described in Chapter 6. Although the terminology is different, in systems terms the overall approach is very similar and broadly compatible. Considering that these two systems approaches were developed in isolation, it is encouraging to find so much common ground.

The CD contains additional details and examples of the Dudley model and further information about approaches to systems and process modelling.

Conclusion

This chapter has sought to show how systems thinking can be applied to the organisational and clinical environment of care pathways. A summary of the ideas behind systems thinking has been provided and this has been related to care pathways. Illustrative examples have shown the relevance of this approach and the potential benefits any one organisation (or health community) can gain from using it.

References

1   Wiener N (1961) *Cybernetics* (2e). MIT Press, Cambridge, MA.
2   Sasieni M, Yaspan A and Friedman L (1959) *Operational Research: methods and problems*. John Wiley, New York.
3   Von Bertalanffy L (1981) General system theory – a critical review. In: Open University Systems Group (eds) *Systems Behaviour* (3e). Open University Press, Buckingham.
4   Beer S (1985) *Diagnosing the System for Organisations*. John Wiley, New York.
5   Forrester JW (1968) *Principles of Systems*. Wright-Allen Press, Cambridge, MA.
6   Checkland P (1981) *Systems Thinking, Systems Practice*. John Wiley, New York.
7   http://www.css.edu/users/dswenson/web/system.htm
8   de Rosnay J (1979) *The Macroscope*. Harper and Row, New York.
9   Secretary of State for Health (2000) *The NHS Plan: a plan for investment, a plan for reform*. (Cm.4818-I.) The Stationery Office, London.
10 Checkland P and Scholes J (1999) *Soft Systems Methodology in Action*. John Wiley, New York.
11 Flood RL and Carson ER (1988) *Dealing with Complexity: an introduction to the theory and application of systems science*. Plenum Press, New York.
12 Forrester JW (1971) Understanding the counterintuitive behaviour of social systems. In: Open University Systems Group (eds) *Systems Behaviour* (3e). Open University Press, Buckingham.
13 Pratt J, Gordon P and Plamping D (1999) *Working Whole Systems*. King's Fund, London.
14 NHS Modernisation Agency (UK) (2002) *Demand Management Group. The Big Wizard*. http://www.demandmanagement.nhs.uk/home.php
15 Wilde G (2002) *A Comparative Evaluation of Process/Service Improvement Techniques*. Dissertation for MBA course, Wolverhampton University. (*See* CD.)
16 http://www.lanner.com/UK/health
17 http://cognitus.co.uk
18 http://www.steyn.dsl.pipex.com/
19 Goldratt EM and Cox J (1993) *The Goal* (2e). Gower, Abingdon.
20 Burton-Houle T (2001) *The Theory of Constraints and its Thinking Processes*. Goldratt Institute, http://www.goldratt.com.
21 Cameron M and Cranfield S (2001) *Managing Change in the NHS: making informed decisions on change*. NCCSDO, School of Hygiene and Tropical Medicine, London, www.sds.lshtm.ac.uk.

22 Davenport TH and Short JE (1990) The new industrial engineering: information technology and business process redesign. *Sloan Management Review*. **Summer**.

23 Hammer M (1990) Reengineering work: don't automate, obliterate. *Harvard Business Review*. **July/August**.

24 Hammer M and Stanton SA (1995) *The Re-engineering Revolution*. Harper Collins, New York.

25 Darnton G and Darnton M (1997) *Business Process Analysis*. International Thompson Business Press, London.

26 Hammer M and Champy J (1993) *Re-engineering the Corporation: a manifesto for business revolution*, p. 74. Nicholas Brealey, London.

27 Mayer RJ *et al.* (1999) *Delivering Results: evolving BPR from art to engineering*, section 1, p. 4. http://www.idef.com/downloads/free_downloads.html. (*See* file bpr art2eng.pdf on CD.)

28 Cancer Services Collaborative (2001) *Redesign: a tool kit*. Hayward Medical Communications, http://www.modern.nhs.uk/improvementguides/process/home.htm.

29 Lathrop JP, Krauss KR and Shows GP (1988) *Operational restructuring – a recipe for success: healthcare viewpoint*. Booz.Allen & Hamilton Inc, McLean, VA.

30 National Institute for Clinical Excellence (2002) *Principles for Best Practice in Clinical Audit*, Figure 1, p. 3. Radcliffe Medical Press, Oxford.

31 Gall J (1986) *Systemantics* (2e). General Systemantics Press, Walker, MN.

32 Lewin K, cited by Spurgeon P and Barwell F (1991) *Implementing Change in the NHS*, p. 46. Chapman & Hall, London in association with HSMC.

33 Department of Health (2000) *National Service Framework for Coronary Heart Disease*. Department of Health, London.

34 Department of Health (2001) *National Service Framework for Older People*. Department of Health, London.

35 http://www.modernnhs.nhs.uk/scripts/default.asp?site_id=21

36 Department of Health (1998) *Information for Health: an information strategy for the modern NHS 1998–2005*. Department of Health, London.

37 http://www.popkin.com

38 http://www.nlm.nih.gov/mesh

39 http://www.cinahl.com

Appendix 5.1: Example diabetic ketoacidosis care pathway

This appendix shows the whole of an example care pathway for treatment of adults with DKA, which was provided courtesy of Dr Newrick, Worcester Acute Hospitals NHS Trust. Additional details are provided on the CD.

Appendix 5.2 shows how example parts of the DKA pathway can be represented in the Dudley care pathway model described in Chapter 5.

DRAFT 6

Worcestershire NHS
Acute Hospitals NHS Trust

Please attach patient sticker here or record:
Name: ....
Unit No: ....
D.O.B: ....
Male   Female

CARE PATHWAY for DIABETIC KETOACIDOSIS (DKA)

To be used for all adults over 16 years with suspicion of or confirmed DKA

This Care Pathway has been developed by a multidisciplinary team. It is intended as a guide to care and treatment, and an aid to documenting patient progress.

All healthcare professionals must exercise their own professional judgment when using this Pathway. However any decision to vary from the Pathway should be documented in the multidisciplinary progress notes to include the reason for variance and action taken.

Any comments regarding this Care Pathway should be directed to Dr P Newrick, Kidderminster Hospital, ext 3383

If you have any problems completing the pathway please contact the Diabetes Specialist Nurses via switch.

Guidelines referred to when developing this Care Pathway:
Guidelines for the management of Diabetic Ketoacidosis. WHAT July 2001
Health Service Ombudsman (2000) Errors in the Care and Treatment of a Young Woman with Diabetes, HMSO, London.
The British Diabetic Association. Diabetes in the UK 1996. British Diabetic Association 1995.
Innes E, Raafat L, Perrin T (2000) Care of Diabetic Ketoacidosis, Clinical Audit and Effectiveness Department WRI NHS TRUST
Textbook of Diabetes. Vol. 1, Chapter 49 pp479-488. Eds. Pickup J and Williams G. Blackwell Scientific Publications

SECTION A - ON ADMISSION: within 1 hour

No.	Desig	INTERVENTION — If an intervention is not carried out for any reason, please tick No and document intervention number, reason and action taken, in multidisciplinary progress notes (Page 5)	Y	N	Signature (and time where appropriate)
1	Dr or RN	Date ...../...../..... Time of admission......... Known diabetes: Yes o No o Type 1 o Type 2 o Insulin Treated Type 2 o Time last took insulin .... Current treatment Previous admissions for DKA Yes o No o Has been vomiting Yes o No o			
2	RN	Nil by Mouth status applied and explained to patient:			
3	RN	Urinalysis for general screening PLUS ketones recorded: *If leukocytes or nitrites present MSU to be sent* Date MSU sent ...../...../..... Ketones present Yes o No o *to be rechecked 12 hourly*			
4	RN	The following observations are recorded: a. Pulse e. Oxygen saturation b. Blood Pressure f. Glasgow coma scale c. Respiratory rate g. Capillary blood glucose d. Temperature			
5	RN	Cardiac monitoring commenced: *ECG if over 50yrs or arrhythmas present* ECG NAD Yes o No o			
6	RN	Fluid balance charting commenced: *hourly if catheterised*			
7	Dr or RN	Blood taken and processed as emergency samples for: a. Full blood count d. Arterial blood pH gases b. Creatinine & Electrolytes e. Blood cultures -*if signs of infection* c. Glucose			
8	Dr	The following interventions considered: *please tick if any are required* Radiology o Cardiac enzymes o Catheterisation o Nasogastric tube o *if drowsy* CVP o *if hypotension, cardiac disease or in the aged*			

9	Dr	DIAGNOSIS:
		DKA o *defined by:*
		    Bicarbonate <16mmols, an elevated glucose and ketonuria ++ or greater
		    or pH < 7.3
		Other o *Exit Care Pathway and record diagnosis in multidisciplinary notes - page 3*
		NB Ketoacidosis can occasionally occur even when plasma glucose is only mildly elevated; it should be excluded by blood gas analysis not by blood glucose alone			

10		Transferred to: HDU o ITU o Other o *All patients should normally go to HDU or ITU. If patient is transferred to another ward please state where and record reason in multidisciplinary notes - page 3* Date and time transferred			
11		Assessed for volume depletion: *Consider CVP* CVP required Yes o No o			
12	Dr	*Administration of bicarbonate is not recommended and only rarely required.* *Seek opinion of senior doctor if bicarbonate is being considered* 20 units Intramuscular soluble insulin prescribed e.g. Actrapid *To be given prior to IV infusion*			
13	Dr	0.9% Normal Saline prescribed as follows: • 1 litre over 30 minutes • 1 litre over 60 minutes • 1 litre over 2 hours Add potassium as required – *see table below*			
14	Dr	IV continuous variable rate infusion of insulin prescribed: *6 units / hr until capillary blood glucose has fallen to less than 10mmols/litre then according to sliding scale 1*			

Potassium Level	Action
> 5.5mmol/l	Do not add potassium
Between 4.5 – 5.5mmol/l	Add 10mmol KCL per litre
4.4mmol/l or less	Add 20 KCL per litre

Capillary blood glucose monitored and recorded hourly and insulin adjusted according to sliding scale 1

Dr = Doctor   RN = Registered Nurse

SECTION C (continued) – Continuing care *within 24 hours of admission*

No.	Desig	INTERVENTION — If an intervention is not carried out for any reason, please tick No and document intervention number, reason and action taken, in multidisciplinary progress notes (Page 5)	Y	N	Signature (and time where appropriate)
27	RN / DSN	**Technique assessed & education given re home urine testing for ketones:**			
28	RN / DSN	**Patient assessed as confident re urine testing for ketones:**			
29	RN / DSN	**Knowledge assessed & educated re illness self management:** Leaflet given – "When you are ill" o			
30	RN / DSN	**Patient assessed as confident re illness self management:**			
31	RN / DSN	**Technique assessed & educated re insulin therapy**			
32	RN / DSN	**Patient assessed as confident re insulin therapy**			

SECTION D – Discharge

33	Dr	**Discharge criteria met / patient fit for discharge:**
		1. Metabolically stable and clinically well
		2. Not vomited within 24 hours
		3. Eating and drinking
		4. Blood sugars less than 20mmols o
		5. Seen by a member of the Diabetes Specialist Team o
		6. Has own blood sugar meter and can use effectively o
		7. Has supply of ketosticks and can use effectively o
		8. Has leaflet "When you are ill" o
		9. Has follow-up appointment with DSN or Diabetologist o
		N.B. Ketonuria alone should not prevent discharge.

Dr = Doctor RN = Registered Nurse DSN = Diabetes Specialist Nurse

Discharged: Date ..../....../......

Following appointment with: Diabetologist: Dr..........................(date) ....../....../......
or   Diabetes Specialist Nurse.................(date) ....../....../......

Signature of Dr discharging patient ....

Please attach patient sticker here or record:
Name:...
Unit No: ....
D.O.B.: ....
Male/Female

SECTION B – Continuing care *within 2 hours of admission*

No.	Desig	INTERVENTION — If an intervention is not carried out for any reason, please tick No and document intervention number, reason and action taken, in multidisciplinary progress notes (Page 5)	Y	N	Signature (and time where appropriate)
16	Dr	**Repeat blood sent 2 hours after initial samples for:** a. Creatinine & Electrolytes b. Glucose c. Arterial blood pH gases			
17	Dr	**Nil By Mouth status reviewed following commencement of treatment:** To remain NBM o Can now eat and drink o *If patient not vomiting and has swallow reflex allow to eat and drink*			
18	Dr	**Further intravenous fluids prescribed:** *Give 3-7 litres over next 20 hours based on assessment of fluid depletion. Consider JVP, urinary output and respiratory function. See criteria for potassium addition page 3 point 9*			
19	Dr	**Prophylactic dose of heparin prescribed:** *If contraindicated please record reason in multidisciplinary notes - page 3*			

Change fluid type to 10% dextrose when capillary blood glucose has fallen to less than 10mmols per litre
Discontinue IV fluids when rehydrated and well enough to eat and drink / discontinue fluid balance charting when IV fluids discontinued

No.	Desig	INTERVENTION	Y	N	Signature
20	RN	**Reassess frequency of monitoring of T, P, R, BP, O2, Sats and GCS:** To be monitored .... hourly			

SECTION C – Continuing care *within 24 hours of admission*

No.	Desig	INTERVENTION	Y	N	Signature
21	Dr	**Repeat blood sent approx 24 hours after initial samples for:** a. Creatinine & Electrolytes b. Glucose			

Convert to subcutaneous insulin when glycaemic control established and well enough to eat and drink.

No.	Desig	INTERVENTION	Y	N	Signature
22	RN	**Referral made to Diabetes Specialist nurse:** *Contact via pager though switch*			
23	Dr or RN	**Referral made to diabetologist:**			
24	Dr	**TTO's prescribed for insulin, hypostop (plus ketosticks if required)**			
25	RN	**Urine checked for ketones 12 hours after admission:** *Continue to check at 12 hourly intervals as long as IV treatment continues*			
26	RN	**Reassess frequency of monitoring of T, P, R, BP O2, Sats and GCS:** To be monitored ....Hourly			

MULTI-DISCIPLINARY PROGRESS NOTES

Please use this sheet to document any additional communications required to ensure appropriate care for patient

No		Sig / Desig Date & Time

DRAFT 6

MULTI-DISCIPLINARY PROGRESS NOTES

Please use this sheet to document any additional communications required to ensure appropriate care for patient

Please attach patient sticker here or record:

Name: ....

Unit No: ....

D.O.B: ....

Male   Female

No		Sig / Desig Date & Time

Appendix 5.2: Example care pathway in *Systems Architect*

This appendix shows an example of how the *Systems Architect* symbolic modelling software will be used in Dudley to capture all the detail required to computerise a care pathway, as outlined in the care pathway definition in Figure 5.7. The example is based on the DKA pathway from Worcester Royal Infirmary, shown in Appendix 5.1. The treatment of the DKA pathway below can be directly compared with the analysis of the same pathway in Chapter 6, Figure 6.3a–d.

Note that this appendix only shows example elements from the whole pathway, which are based on a 'reading' of the paper pathway. Any clinical elements included or excluded in the example are therefore the responsibility of the author of this chapter, not the pathway team from Worcester.

In practice, a local care pathway development team would devise their own process maps and agree the content of process steps and tasks with the support of a facilitator. The diagrams and definitions would be entered into *Systems Architect* by the facilitator and published for review via the intranet (*see* Figure 5.5).

The starting point for the care pathway model is a process map, shown in Figure 5A2.1. Since DKA is an acute medical problem with relatively clear diagnostic test results, the high-level process map for the pathway is linear, with stages leading from a confirmed diagnosis, to treatment, to discharge, to follow-up. Optional investigations and treatments within the pathway are stored at lower levels in the pathway model.

The three dots above the stage 'initial treatment' indicate that there is a 'child diagram' linked to that stage. This is a process chart, shown in Figure 5A2.2. The process chart for this stage is divided into three

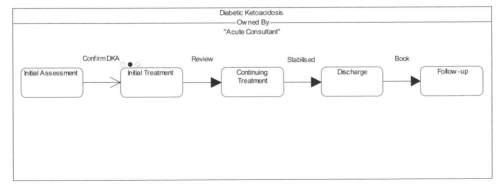

Figure 5A2.1   DKA pathway process map.

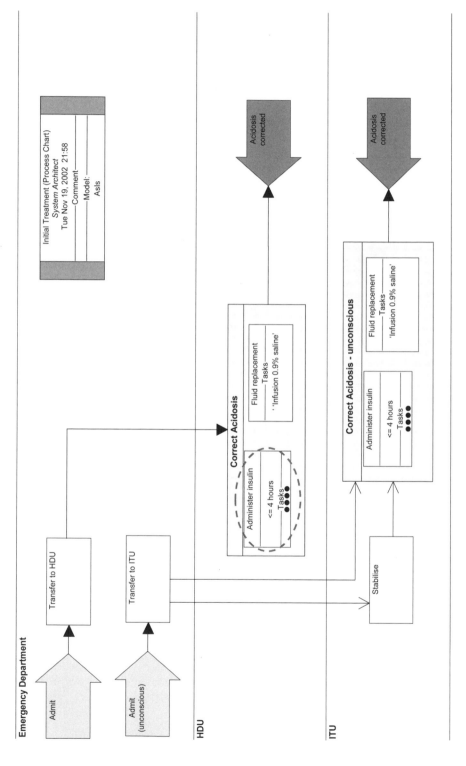

Figure 5A2.2 Process chart for 'initial treatment' stage (dotted oval highlights process step covered in Figure 5A2.3).

horizontal bands or 'swim-lanes'. These show which departments are responsible for specific process steps – emergency department, high dependency unit (HDU) and intensive therapy unit (ITU).

The main clinical objective of the initial treatment stage is to restore glucose and fluid levels to within normal range. More severely affected patients will be treated in ITU, where additional or different treatment may be required to stabilise the patient. Optional paths are shown by the lines with open arrowheads. In practice, some of the initial treatment may be carried out in the emergency department before transfer to HDU or ITU – this would be a matter for local agreement and is not shown on the example process chart.

In the DKA pathway, administration of intravenous insulin and fluids is continued until test results show that glucose and fluid levels (and possibly other variables such as potassium) are within their normal range. The two main process steps – administer insulin and fluid replacement – are therefore contained within a shaded box labelled 'correct acidosis', which in this type of diagram represents an 'iteration'. This means that all the activities within the box are continued until specific conditions are met.

The process step 'administer insulin' is highlighted with a dotted oval. This is not a standard symbol on process charts, but is used here to indicate which process step is described in more detail below. By selecting the process step from a list, or by double-clicking on the symbol on the diagram, its definition can be displayed.

Figure 5A2.3a–e show typical forms used within *System Architect* to define process steps and the tasks within them. These data are held within the encyclopaedia and can be exported, in whole or part, in a number of formats. Note that additional forms (as well as the diagrams above) are used to define a care pathway and its stages. The pathway definition can be developed and adapted over time because the content and layout of all these forms can be tailored by editing a configuration file for each encyclopaedia. It is possible to change the configuration of an encyclopaedia, even when it already contains data.

The process step definition is displayed in several tabbed forms, including 'Clinical Attributes' as shown in Figure 5A2.3a and b. Each tab can have one or more pages – in this case there are two. Very few of the entries on the forms are mandatory – the detail required for a complete definition can therefore be built up gradually and may not be available or relevant for some process steps.

The 'Tasklist' tab shown in Figure 5A2.3c is a summary list of tasks within the process step. New tasks can be added easily using the 'insert' and 'choices' buttons. The full encyclopaedia will contain a catalogue of standard investigative tests and therapies to ensure that all pathways use the same definitions for this type of task. A matching set will also be set up within the EPR system.

Clicking on a specific task brings up additional forms for the full task definition – examples are shown in Figure 5A2.3d and e.

It is therefore possible in *Systems Architect* to traverse the full range of the care pathway definition in Figure 5.7 with just a few mouse-clicks and to progressively build up the detail required for a computerised care pathway. This detailed view is maintained in the encyclopaedia independently of the method used to implement the pathway.

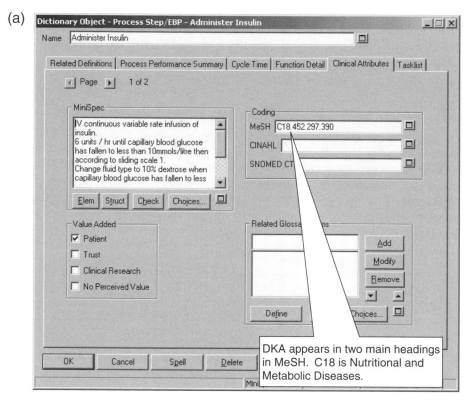

Figure 5A2.3 (a) and (b) Example process step definition forms in *Systems Architect*. (c) Example process step definition form – task list. (d) and (e) Example task definition forms (blood test).

(b)

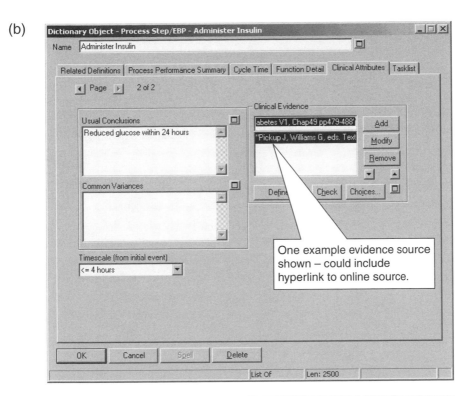

One example evidence source shown – could include hyperlink to online source.

(c)

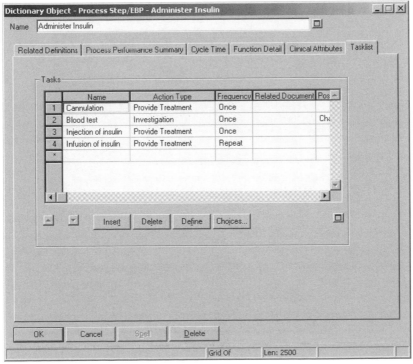

(d)

(e)

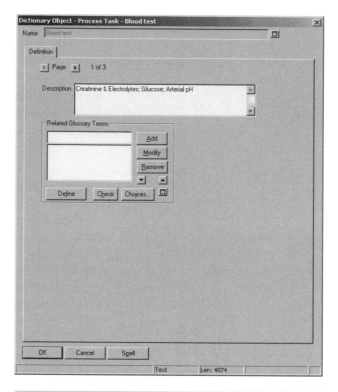

6

Developing e-pathway standards

Ruth Page and Ian Herbert

Key points

- There is urgent need for standardisation of definitions and concepts relating to care pathways.

- It is possible (and necessary) to differentiate between the similar concepts of care pathways, guidelines and protocols.

- A conceptual structure for care pathways is proposed which could provide the necessary standardisation to enable software designers to build computer modules to support the development of e-pathways.

Introduction

The purpose of this chapter is to explain why a standardised set of definitions is needed to describe care pathways and related (but different) concepts, and why this is an essential requirement for the successful development of e-pathways. The chapter goes on to describe what we will call here a *Care Pathway Conceptual Structure*, which aims to model the relationships between concepts and offer definitions which could become standards. The Care Pathway Conceptual Structure is illustrated with the use of an example care pathway.

Why model?

The previous chapter describes the concept of a care pathway as a model. It focuses on the act of a multidisciplinary team agreeing on an ideal patient journey from which to guide (and benchmark) what happens in reality. It takes a systems approach, and considers the effect of care pathways on an organisation and their application as a way of redesigning processes within healthcare.

Historically, care pathways have been developed and used locally by a ward, a department or organisation. As long as the people using the care pathways understood the intended use, and the care pathway was used accordingly, then there was no issue regarding what was being represented. What happened outside the pathway's remit did not matter. There was not a need for standardisation beyond their own boundaries, and certainly not at a national level. But the NHS information strategy, *Information for Health* (1998),[1] in 1998, implied that electronic patient records should be structured by care pathways, across organisational boundaries when necessary, and made the need for national standard specifications and definitions very clear.

The NHS Information Authority[2] (NHSIA) and Information Policy Unit[3] can propose national standards for system specifications and data definitions to the NHS Information Standards Board. The NHS is required to follow approved standards. If it does not, then it will not be possible to understand the inputs or outputs of an electronic system, or to share data, transmit messages or aggregate and analyse data on any scale other than the local. This applies both to the knowledge represented in care pathways and the results of their application to individual patient care. It would be impossible to know if something meant the same from one system to the next. What is more, the standards need to be sufficiently detailed and unambiguous so that computer software can interpret data conforming to them. If this is so, then it will become possible to move towards computer-based clinical decision support and work-flow management. Without standardisation of concepts and definitions, software designers will have no consistency on which to base their designs of computer modules to support the use of e-pathways.

At present even the expression 'care pathway' means a multitude of things to many people, and makes it impossible to know for certain what is being described. The lack of concepts and definitions which are universally understood and accepted has been outlined in Chapter 1. It has already been argued that the confusion in terminology and definitions impedes the speed of development of care pathways and wastes staff time trying to clarify their understanding of different but related concepts.

The expression 'care pathway' commonly includes a more general description of a patient journey or high-level process mapping of services and packages of care. It is also used for concepts with purposes similar to care pathways that aid decision making and treatment, such as guidelines and protocols. But all of these uses do not have exactly the same meaning or intention, thus making it difficult to interpret or use the expression 'care pathway' in a consistent way.

There is a tendency for healthcare specialists using guidelines, protocols, work-flows, care pathways etc. to explain the processes within this similar family of concepts from a single point of view. There are organisations that have implemented guidelines; others, care pathways; others, protocols. Each has much to offer in explaining, mapping and recording the care and decision making of care provision, but it is an assumption to think of them all as meaning the same, or that one concept on its own covers such processes comprehensively.

Care pathways, protocols and guidelines are all essentially a 'path' of sorts. All of them have the aim of supporting effective regimens of care. But each concept operates differently, enough to merit being a separate concept with a distinct approach and purpose. It is necessary to draw distinctions between these and other similar concepts for a number of reasons. In order to model the processes using the concepts, electronically or otherwise, there needs to be one standard definition for each concept that is clear and concise. The use and purpose of the concepts within systems of care provision need to be consistent. Being clear about the distinctions between concepts would provide a standard language so that clinicians, health informatics specialists, system suppliers and others can reliably refer to the concepts and exchange instances of them. The definitions we have adopted are as follows:

- **clinical guideline** – 'systematically developed statements to assist practitioner and patient decisions about appropriate healthcare for specific clinical circumstances'[4]
- **clinical protocol** – agreed statements with explicit steps based on clinical guidelines and/or organisational consensus. The agreement is binding for a specified community, which may be a team or larger organisation. The clinical protocol may say which kind of care professional can perform an action, or even name a specific individual as an action's performer. It can be for a single discipline (as can a guideline)

- **care pathway** – a structured document that:
  - identifies the actions to do/not to do appropriate to the health issue it is for. It is likely to include actions recommended by one (or more) protocol and guideline, and should include those to be performed by all the staff disciplines involved. A care pathway may also indicate any constraints on the staff discipline that may perform a specific activity (and may name the individual who should perform it)
  - contains goals and the sequence of actions specific to the health issue
  - will be used to record the care provided for that issue, its outcomes and other information about the state of individual patients to whom it is applied
  - evolves, subject to version control, according to the outcomes of its use and advances in clinical practice and technology.

Given the definitions above, we need to go further and create a standardised conceptual structure for care pathways. Without such a structure it will not be possible to achieve a generic specification for electronic systems. This structure is needed nationally to inform developments in the Healthcare Records Infrastructure programme, and other programmes of work to develop clinical computer systems, including EPR, EHR and the more recent draft for an Integrated Care Record System (ICRS). (The EPR and EHR concepts have been described previously in Chapter 4.)

History

Efforts towards achieving standard definitions and use of care pathways have been going on for some time. In the UK, work on establishing criteria for care pathways began with the mental health subgroup of the National Pathways Association[5] (NPA) in 1999. The group wanted to have a collection of care pathways used in mental health to be available to others as reference material. A standard set of criteria was deemed necessary to ensure that the care pathways intended for this library were indeed care pathways and not something else called a care pathway. All too frequently, examples of protocols or guidelines were called care pathways but did not meet the criteria.

Taking on this task was considered not possible by some people, based on the thinking that there were too many views about what constituted a care pathway; but the group persevered. Consensus was reached, and it was felt that the criteria developed were in fact appropriate for any care pathway, not just those for mental health.

The initial criteria were placed on the NPA website for comment.

Feedback suggested that the criteria were quite useful, particularly for organisations that were developing pathways for the first time. Being part of the origins of this work, these criteria have been included in the additional information contained on the CD.

The NHSIA has been analysing clinical computer systems developed by NHS trusts for electronic care pathway application and their potential for general applicability across the NHS. To do this, a standard structure with set concepts, definitions for each and an understanding of how they work together was necessary. It was this challenge that led to the development of the Care Pathway Conceptual Structure. Once the model was conceived and concepts specifically defined and understood, it was then possible to interpret care pathway activity in someone else's system.

The Care Pathway Conceptual Structure was tested against real systems as part of the development process. This not only gave us a way to interpret how care pathway concepts were being applied, it also proved to be a good test for the model. The basic question being asked was: 'Did the Care Pathway Conceptual Structure include everything at sample sites?' It was through this testing process that much was revealed about the concepts and what constituted a comprehensive care pathway definition.

Independently, from 1992, members of the Healthcare Modelling Programme at the NHS Information Management Centre were working with clinicians to model clinical guidelines. This work was part of two pan-European initiatives, DILEMMA[6] and PRESTIGE,[7] which were designing and piloting computer software to support guideline authoring and use. The team incorporated results of the collaboration into the NHS Healthcare Model, a generalised business model of healthcare that they had been working on for some time. The Care Pathway Conceptual Structure presented in this chapter is based on the NHS Healthcare Model.

What are we modelling?

There are many kinds of models. Each is characterised by what is being modelled, and how it is done. Our purpose here is to define the kinds of information that care pathway definitions contain, the information that results from their use and the associations between these two aspects of care pathways in order to:

- provide a common, understandable language for the electronic interchange of care pathways as *knowledge*
- enable the results of using them for patient care to be electronically interchanged, aggregated and analysed without loss of meaning
- make both kinds of data amenable to computation, so that software can

be built to comprehensively support care pathway authors, users and those analysing the variances that results from their use. Paper-based pathways impose artificial constraints because they suggest a fixed content and temporal sequence. Computerisation frees us from the tyranny of the form (which, however, does have advantages that we should be careful not to lose).

We are not concerned here with any particular care pathway, or any one organisation's approach to using them. The intention is to provide general-purpose information structures which can accommodate all the knowledge in any care pathway, and which cater for the use of care pathways in any circumstances, including multidisciplinary, multi-provider settings. The Care Pathway Conceptual Structure proposed in this chapter is not designed specifically for computer systems, but rather is a business information model that is the essential foundation for the design of such systems.

The following tasks were identified as important stages in developing the Care Pathway Conceptual Structure:

- Identify the life cycle of a care pathway as a piece of knowledge that is authored.
- Identify the separate life cycle of a care pathway when it is used to guide care delivery for a particular problem for a specific patient.
- Determine which concepts are components of care pathways.
- Determine which concepts are processes within care pathways.
- Decide on the scope of concepts that are within the care pathway system.
- Determine which concepts are so similar that they are synonyms of others.
- Define concepts based on a literature search and examples practised in the UK.
- Build the structure based on the concepts, their properties and the relationships between them. The modelling used the Unified Modelling Language (UML), which is the standard modelling language used in the NHSIA for this sort of purpose.

The main concepts in the Care Pathway Conceptual Structure

The Care Pathway Conceptual Structure proposed in this chapter covers the expected treatment and care for patients who have a particular health issue, the actual outcomes of this care and any variance that occurs during the time the patient is on the care pathway. Included are concepts that relate to:

- development (i.e. 'authoring') of a care pathway
- links between the knowledge in a pathway and the evidence supporting it
- the activities and interventions that are expected to happen as part of the care pathway, those that are planned for an individual patient in their care plan and those that are actually delivered
- the information to be recorded about the patient and the health issue specified for a care pathway
- variations in one or more categories, including the interventions that are carried out, who does what, the outcome for the patient, and other information recorded about the patient.

The conceptual structure distinguishes between two major components:

- the Model Care Pathway
- the Care Pathway Use.

Each has a set of states which make up its life cycle, and different qualities and purposes. These are outlined below and shown schematically in Figure 6.1. In the text we distinguish the component parts of the conceptual structure by using a different typeface – thus.

The Model Care Pathway represents a structured piece of knowledge that describes how to care for a specific health issue. It has an overall objective that explains the intention of the care pathway, and is related to the characteristics demonstrated by a particular group of patients plus the signs and symptoms associated with the health issue. Activities and interventions, when they should take place and by whom, are specified in the Model Care Pathway as it forms the template for clinical staff to later apply to individual patients. The Model Care Pathway is the main outcome of the work of a Care Pathway Development Team.

A Care Pathway Use is a Model Care Pathway that is being (or has been) applied to a specific patient and health issue, and includes the patient-related data gathered as a result. It allows for individuality when applying the Model Care Pathway to a patient. It is possible to record other signs and symptoms that are pertinent to the health issue for an individual patient that may not be specified in the Model Care Pathway. Activities or interventions can also be individualised for the patient as well as specific patient outcomes. If interventions are delayed, done differently or not at all, these variations can be captured.

A Care Pathway Use in the 'ended' state explains on what basis the patient left the care pathway, in addition to being a closed record of care

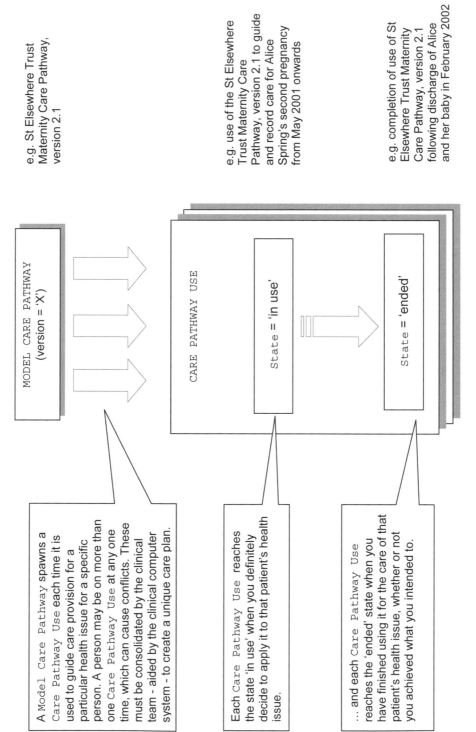

Figure 6.1 Main concepts in the Care Pathway Conceptual Structure.

for an individual patient. It can then be used for clinical audit and analysis.

The flexibility provided by the distinction between the Model Care Pathway and the Care Pathway Use for a specific patient addresses one of the major clinical concerns that pathways are healthcare-by-numbers. Although the Care Pathway Conceptual Structure is abstract and could in principle apply to paper or computerised care pathways, in practice only the latter can provide this high degree of flexibility.

Care pathway conceptual structure: overview

An overview of the Care Pathway Conceptual Structure is described below. This overview introduces the major concepts and sets the scene for the more detailed explanation given on the accompanying CD. On the CD there are more detailed information and diagrams from the Care Pathway Conceptual Structure.

The Care Pathway Conceptual Structure has been developed using a standard approach to describing information systems, known as the Unified Modelling Language.[8,9] A brief, less technical explanation of UML diagramming conventions is given below. The *System Architect* modelling tool described in Chapter 5 was used to draw the UML diagrams. The advantage of UML in this context is that it is standardised, well understood by IT professionals and suppliers, independent of how the model is implemented in software, and can be used as a starting point for software design. More broadly, UML is being used by the NHSIA in a range of contexts, so that over time a consistent framework for NHS information systems is being developed.

UML is a very rich way of specifying information systems using what is known as an 'object-oriented approach'. UML models include three fundamental elements – things, relationships and diagrams. UML is therefore a symbolic modelling language in the sense described in Chapter 5. In the Care Pathway Conceptual Structure we are concerned mainly with structural things (nouns), in particular what are known as 'classes'. A class is a detailed description of a set of objects which share attributes, behaviour and relationships (with other classes). UML classes mirror the system being modelled, thus at the centre of the Care Pathway Conceptual Structure we find the class Patient.

Figure 6.2 is the high-level overview of the Care Pathway Conceptual Structure. In this diagram, the rectangular boxes with names in capitals are 'classes'. They represent the concept named in capital letters in the box. The words in the lower part of each class box represent 'attributes'.

Attributes are the details about the class concept represented in the box that are important to know. In this example, the class Model Care Pathway has attributes of version ID, review date and version description.

In Figure 6.2 the key in the top-right corner summarises the conventions that:

- Shaded boxes represent the concepts to be found in the Model Care Pathway (and Model Care Pathway Core, which holds the small amount of information which does not vary from version to version of the pathway). This is the care pathway that has been agreed and authorised by the organisation or group of clinicians that use it and includes references to the clinical guidelines and protocols used for guiding treatment and care, and the documentation structure for recording care. In a paper implementation, it is the equivalent of the master copy of the (unused) care pathway forms. Note that each version of the Model Care Pathway is distinct.
- Unshaded classes represent the Care Pathway Use, i.e. the Model Care Pathway (version) when activated for a specific patient. It is the working document and care pathway for an individual patient. In paper terms, it represents the care pathway forms bearing the patient's name, address and other demographic details, and which hold progressively more data about that patient's care as the use of the care pathway proceeds. When completed it becomes the patient's clinical record for the health issue that the pathway is dealing with.

The Patient class is highlighted by a box with a thick black line round it, because it represents a type of person which is different from the other concepts (note that this is not standard UML notation). The other boxes with dotted edges contain notes that provide more detail and explanation of the classes.

Solid black lines linking boxes show that there is a relationship between classes. The relationship is described very briefly with the words in italics located along the lines. For example:

a Care Pathway Use *(is) for care of* Patient

This simply means that a single Care Pathway Use is used to guide and record the care of a particular patient, or to put it another way, each application of the Model Care Pathway to a patient's health issue creates a Care Pathway Use.

The dashed lines between classes represent variance and depict the potential differences between what is expected as given in the model care pathway and what really happens when the pathway is used for a patient and becomes a Care Pathway Use.

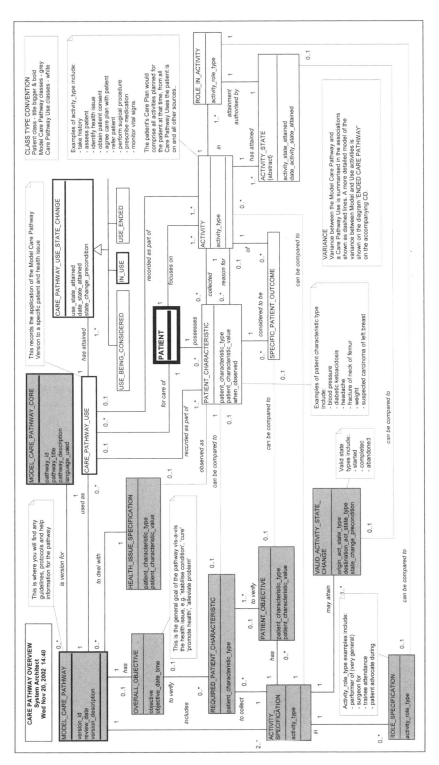

Figure 6.2 Care Pathway Conceptual Structure overview.

Knowing how many of one class (or concept) can occur as it relates to another class is an important feature in modelling as it helps to explain the relationships between them. This is known as 'cardinality' and is represented in the model by 0..* (0 to many), 1 (only 1), 1..* (one to many) and 0..1 (none or one). To give an example, in the overview, one `Model Care Pathway` can have no version or one or many versions. This is shown in the map by 0..* on the line labelled *'is version for'*. Though it is always good practice to use version control, the fact that it is still possible to have a `Model Care Pathway` in its early stages of development without version details has been included to be as comprehensive as possible in modelling real practice.

This basic description of UML modelling explains the lines and boxes of Figure 6.2 and helps to relate the concepts. The diagram may appear complex, but it is included here to show how precisely defined concepts can be assembled to provide a standardised definition of 'care pathway' which is suitable for specification and implementation of clinical computer systems which support e-pathways. A full set of definitions that includes every class of the detailed Care Pathway Conceptual Structure is on the CD.

To illustrate how these abstract concepts can be applied, the next section shows how elements of a real care pathway can be related back to the classes and attributes in the Care Pathway Conceptual Structure.

Using a real example: the diabetic ketoacidosis care pathway

To demonstrate how the Care Pathway Conceptual Structure works in practice, a sample model care pathway on DKA has been supplied by Worcester Acute Hospitals NHS Trust.[10] The same sample care pathway was used to illustrate the Dudley healthcare community's care pathway model described in Chapter 5. The complete DKA care pathway is attached as an appendix to Chapter 5 and is also available on the CD.

In this chapter, sections of the care pathway are shown with classes from the Care Pathway Conceptual Structure superimposed (*see* Figure 6.3a–d). A brief description of these classes is given below each section of the sample DKA care pathway to help explain their use.

In general, it is only possible to show in Figure 6.3 the classes that are present in the `Model Care Pathway`, as the care pathway would need to be 'in use' or 'ended' for a specific patient to show the other classes specific to a `Care Pathway Use`. However, some of the other classes

Continued on p. 170

Figure 6.3   DKA sample pathway relationship to Care Pathway Conceptual Structure (a)–(d).

(a)

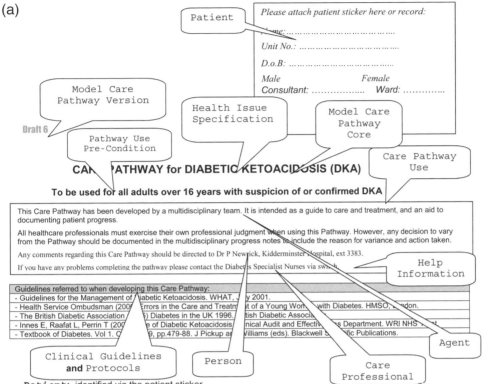

Patient: identified via the patient sticker.
Model Care Pathway: identified by the version number.
Model Care Pathway Core: title identifies that this is a Model Care Pathway for DKA. This information cannot change from version to version.
Health Issue Specification: the condition for which this is a Model Care Pathway. Again this cannot change from version to version.
[Pathway Use Pre-Condition]: a pre-condition for entering the care pathway.
Care Pathway Use: This care pathway is the chosen means for guiding care and treatment of DKA in this Trust.
[Agent]: a person or body of people who act purposefully and make decisions, for example, the multi-disciplinary pathway authoring team.
[Person]: a named individual, i.e. the name of the lead clinician to contact regarding the care pathway.
[Care Professional]: a specific professional.
[Help Information]: help information details.
[Clinical Guidelines & Protocols]: references given that support interventions within care pathway, and on which its content is based.

(b)

2	RN	**Nil by Mouth status applied and explained to patient:**		
3	RN	**Urinalysis for general screening PLUS ketones recorded:** *If leukocytes or nitrites present MSU to be sent* Date MSU sent ....../....../...... Ketones present Yes ❏ No ❏ *to be rechecked 12 h......*		
4	RN	**The following observations are recorded:** a. Pulse e. Oxygen saturation b. Blood pressure f. Glasgow coma scale c. Respiratory rate g. Capillary blood glucose d. Temperature		

> Required Patient Characteristic

Required Patient Characteristics: observations and clinical findings that should be recorded.

(c)

> Role Specification

> Activity Variance

> Activity Specification

> Valid Activity State

No.	Design	**INTERVENTION** If an intervention is not carried out for any reason, please tick 'No' and document intervention number, reason and action taken, in multi-disciplinary progress notes (page 5).	Y	N	**Signature** (and time where appropriate)
16	Dr	**Repeat blood sent 2 hours after initial samples for:** a. Creatinine & electrolytes b. Glucose c. Arterial blood pH gases			
17	Dr	**Nil By Mouth status reviewed for treatment:** To remain NBM ❏ Can now eat and drink ❏ *If patient not vomiting and has swallow reflex allow to eat and drink.*			
18	Dr	**Further intravenous fluids prescribed:** *Give 3-7 litres over next 20 hours based on assessment of fluid depletion. Consider JVP, urinary output and respiratory function. See criteria for potassium addition - page 3, point 9.*			
19	Dr	**Prophylactic dose of heparin prescribed:** *If contraindicated please record reason in multidisciplinary notes - page 3.*			

Change fluid type to 10% dextrose when capillary blood glucose has fallen to less than 10 mmol per litre. Discontinue IV fluids when rehydrated and well enough to eat and drink / discontinue fluid balance charting when IV fluids discontinued.

[Activity Variance]: one type of variance. Any variance or alteration in delivering care that is different from the specified activity in the Model Care Pathway.
Activity Specification: the activities or interventions as specified in the Model Care Pathway.
Role Specification: the designated role that is required by an intervention as stated in the Model Care Pathway.
Valid Activity State: certain conditions must be present in order to proceed. Interventions may have a particular start date and time, or be dependent on another intervention taking place first, or the patient needs to be in a particular state in order to proceed.

(d)

Abandoned Care Pathway Use

9	Dr	**DIAGNOSIS:** DKA ❑ *defined by:* *Bicarbonate <16 mmol, an elevated glucose and ketonuria ++ or greater* *or pH < 7.3* Other ❑ *Exit Care Pathway and record diagnosis in multidisciplinary notes - page 3* NB: Ketoacidosis can occasionally occur even when plasma glucose is only mildly elevated; it should be excluded by blood gas analysis not by blood glucose alone.

Overall Objective

33	Dr	**Discharge criteria met/patient fit for discharge:** 1. Metabolically stable and clinically well ❑ 2. Not vomited within 24 hours ❑ 3. Eating and drinking ❑ 4. Blood sugars less than 20 mmol ❑ 5. Seen by a member of the Diabetes Specialist Team ❑ 6. Has own blood sugar meter and can use effectively ❑ 7. Has supply of ketosticks and can use effectively ❑ 8. Has leaflet 'When you are ill' ❑ 9. Has follow-up appointment with DSN or diabetologist ❑ *NB: Ketonuria alone should not prevent discharge.*

Patient Objective

Discharged: Date ..../............./...............

Following appointment with: Diabetologist: Dr...

(date)   ...../...../.....   *or*

                                           Diabetes Specialist Nurse............................

(date)   ...../...../.....

Role Specification

Signature of Dr discharging patient: ....

[Abandoned Care Pathway Use]: the patient is taken off the care pathway before completing the care pathway in its entirety.
Overall Objective: the main intention to be achieved for the patient.
Patient Objective: a specific patient objective that relates to a set of interventions.
Role Specification: a role that someone – the Actor – must perform in an activity.
Actor tells you who or what type of person should perform the role.

from the complete Care Pathway Conceptual Structure can also be included in the diagrams below because they are represented in the sample DKA care pathway. These classes are identified with square brackets [. . .] around them in the brief descriptions below each diagram.

Appendix 6.1 shows a table where the DKA model care pathway is more completely mapped to the classes in the Care Pathway Conceptual Structure overview and the more detailed diagrams on the CD. Examples of instances and explanations are given for those classes that cover a care pathway 'in use' and 'ended'. By referring to the example extracts in Figure 6.3 and the complete sample pathway in Chapter 5, the full relationship between the Care Pathway Conceptual Structure and a real pathway can be visualised.

To illustrate how the Care Pathway Conceptual Structure relates to the 'model' DKA pathway, we look below at who does what and when for which objectives, and the activity variances.

The classes that describe the *who* are [Agent], [Person], [Care Professional], Role Specification, Actor and Patient. In this example, the care pathway clearly states that the multidisciplinary team is the Agent (a person or group of people who act purposefully) that has developed the DKA Model Care Pathway. A Person is a named individual. Any comments regarding this care pathway are to be directed to the doctor whose name is given on the care pathway document. A Care Professional is a role played by a Person, an Agent whose business it is to provide care. In the example care pathway, the diabetes specialist nurse is listed as the care professional to contact for assistance. Actor and Role Specification are well depicted at the end of the care pathway, where the doctor (the Actor Specification) responsible (the Role Specification) for discharging the patient from the care pathway signs the care pathway. This indicates what type of professional should perform a particular role, that of discharging the patient. A Patient is a person who is in the role of receiving (but involved) in his or her own care.

What the care pathway is about is described by the Health Issue Specification for a care pathway, by a [Pathway Use Pre-Condition], the Required Patient Characteristics, the Activity Specification, the [Guidelines and Protocols] that support this, and the title and version of the Model Care Pathway. These classes are clearly visible on the example care pathway. As often happens, the Health Issue Specification (the patient state or condition) is incorporated into the title of the care pathway, followed by the precondition that it is for all adults over the age of 16. The Required Patient Characteristics – the signs and symptoms to be addressed – add to the information gathered for this health issue. What is to be done according to the interventions in the care pathway are specified as `Activity Specification` and based on the guidelines and protocols adopted by the trust.

When activities or interventions are to be done is given in the `Valid Activity State` (typically what needs to be true in order to start an intervention). The care pathway example is very explicit in guiding the user as to when to start an intervention, whether it be within the first hour, within two hours of admission or 24 hours. There are also numerous interventions that need a certain precondition to be present before starting them, i.e. 'change fluid type to 10% glucose when capillary blood glucose has fallen to less than 10 mmols per litre'.

Which objectives are addressed at two distinct levels. One – `Overall Objective` – focuses on the overall purpose or intention of the care pathway. The other – `Patient Objective` – is more specific to the patient and a particular intervention within the pathway, and is about achieving an improvement in their symptoms. Both of these are explicitly demonstrated in this example care pathway. The purpose or intention is to stabilise the patient's condition, and more specifically, to 'not vomit within 24 hours, to be eating and drinking, and for the patient to have blood sugars less than 20 mmol'.

Activity variance, which is one type of variance, is clearly identified in the example care pathway. On each page of the care pathway that lists interventions, a clause is written that explains how to record the reason why and other action taken against an intervention that is not carried out. The Care Pathway Conceptual Structure also includes variance for other things in addition to differences in interventions. These include a change in the role from what type of care professional carries out an intervention from that specified, differences in activity states as to when something is done, differences between patient objectives and specific patient outcomes, and differences in the patient characteristics, or signs and symptoms recorded against what it is required to record.

Other related work on care pathways from the NHS Information Authority

The major work elsewhere on care pathways within the NHS Information Authority is being carried out by the National electronic Library for Health in conjunction with the Royal College of Nursing (RCN). The NeLH launched a national Care Pathways Database in 2001.[11] It contains listings of over 2000 pathways currently in use, and full text versions of over 100. Work is under way to:

- rationalise the database indexing, nomenclature and classification
- cross-link it to other NeLH resources, such as the NeLH guidelines database
- explore national arrangements for appraisal, and electronic sharing of pathways.

The pathways can be browsed in alphabetic order by pathway title, topic, source organisation and user site. The database contains the status of each pathway, plus contact details for those wishing to find out more about it, and an associated full-text search tool.

Other work on care pathways took place at several sites within the recently completed Electronic Record Development and Implementation Programme (ERDIP). Readers should consult the ERDIP website[12] for further details: a single document summarising the ERDIP work on care pathways is not currently available.

Conclusion

This chapter has explained why standardised definitions and a common understanding of distinct but related concepts is so important for the future development of e-pathways. The confusion around terminology and definitions has already been a hindrance to care pathway development and this situation will get worse in a computerised environment if different care pathway computer modules are developed which interpret concepts differently. A Care Pathway Conceptual Structure developed in Unified Modelling Language has been proposed which attempts to provide this standardisation. The process of developing the Care Pathway Conceptual Structure and testing it against sample care pathways has itself clarified the relationship between multiple concepts in this field of knowledge.

References

1 Department of Health (1998) *Information for Health: an information strategy for the modern NHS 1998–2005*. Department of Health, London.
2 NHS Information Authority, http://www.nhsia.nhs.uk.
3 Department of Health Information Policy Unit, http://www.doh.gov.uk/ipu/index.htm.
4 Field MJ and Lohr KN (eds) (1992) *Guidelines for Clinical Practice*. National Academy Press, Washington, DC.

5   National Pathways Association (NPA), http://www.the-npa.org.
6   DILEMMA Project, http://www.acl.icnet.uk/lab/dilemma.html.
7   PRESTIGE Project, http://www.rbh.nthames.nhs.uk/prestige/index.htm.
8   Booch G, Rumbaugh J and Jacobson I (1999) *The Unified Modelling Language User Guide.* Addison Wesley, Reading, MA.
9   Eriksson HE and Penker M (2000) *Business Modelling with UML: business patterns at work.* John Wiley & Sons, New York.
10 Newrick P *et al. Care Pathway for Diabetic Ketoacidosis (DKA): draft version 6.* Worcester Acute Hospitals NHS Trust.
11 National electronic Library for Health Care Pathways Database, http://www.nelh.nhs.uk/carepathways.asp.
12 Electronic Record Development and Implementation Programme (ERDIP), http://www.nhsia.nhs.uk/erdip/pages/default.asp.

Appendix 6.1: Detailed mapping of DKA pathway to the Care Pathway Conceptual Structure

The table on the following pages provides a more complete list of how the components within the sample DKA care pathway can be represented in the Care Pathway Conceptual Structure.

References to classes are shown in title-case `Courier Font`, and to class attributes in lower-case `courier font`.

Care pathway element from the DKA example . . .	*. . . is represented in the model as*
Stated in care pathway: Care Pathway for Diabetic Ketoacidosis (DKA)	`Model Care Pathway Core`
Stated: Version 6 'Review Date' – space in footer of document	`Model Care Pathway`
Stated: 'Draft'	`Model Care Pathway State`
Stated: Diagnosis not DKA 'Diagnosis: other – exit care pathway and record diagnosis in multidisciplinary notes'	`state change precondition` for the 'abandoned' state of the `Model Care Pathway`
Stated: Diabetic Ketoacidosis (DKA) Diagnosis: DKA if bicarbonate < 16 mmol, an elevated glucose and ketonuria ++ or greater, or pH <7.3	`Health Issue Specification` for the `Model Care Pathway Core` The **detailed definition of DKA** would appear in the `state change precondition` for the 'Use Being Considered' state
Stated: All adults over 16 years	`state change precondition` for the 'Use being considered' state of the `Model Care Pathway`

Stated: 'patient fit for discharge' and meets discharge criteria – general intentions to be achieved for the patient	Overall Objective of the Model Care Pathway
Explanation: Within the trust's local guidelines document, details are given for assessment, criteria for diagnosis and treatment, i.e. sliding scale insulin – these are protocols	Clinical Protocol(s) for the Model Care Pathway
Stated: Section included in care pathway on 'guidelines referred to when developing this care pathway'	Clinical Guideline(s) for the Model Care Pathway
Stated: 'If you have any problems completing the pathway please contact the Diabetes Specialist Nurse via switch'	Help Information
Examples in care pathway: Pulse, BP, respiratory rate, temperature, oxygen saturation, Glasgow coma scale, capillary blood glucose Urinalysis for general screening plus ketones recorded	Required Patient Characteristic(s)
Ex: To be able to eat and drink (patient objective) 'Nil by mouth status reviewed following commencement of treatment' (activity specification), 'if patient is not vomiting and has swallow reflex (*patient objectives*) allow to eat and drink'. The patient objective would be that the patient is 'now able to eat and drink'	Patient Objective for related Activity Specification
	This caters for all patient objectives that relate to particular interventions, i.e. Activity Specification(s)
Ex: 'Nil by mouth', 'Cardiac monitoring', 'Fluid balance monitoring', 'Blood taken and processed', 'assessed for volume depletion', 'referral made to diabetologist'	Activity Specification(s)
Ex: Start 'nasogastric tube if drowsy', 'consider CVP if hypotension, cardiac disease or in the aged'	'is drowsy' would be 'start' state change precondition for Activity Specification 'use nasogastric tube'

Continued

Care pathway element from the DKA example . . .	. . . is represented in the model as
Ex. 'Add potassium as required: if > 5.5 mmol/l, do not add potassium between 4.5–5.5 mmol/l, add 10 mmol KCL per litre 4.4 mmol/l or less, add 20 KCL per litre'	
Ex: 'Continue to check urine for ketones at 12-hourly intervals as long as IV treatment continues'	'IV treatment started and > 12 hours after last urine check' would be `state change precondition` for 'start' of `Activity Specification` 'check urine for ketones'
Ex: do not add potassium if level is > 5.5 mmol/l	'potassium ≤ 5.5 mmol/l' would be `state change precondition` for 'add potassium' `Activity Specification`
Stated: RN, DSN, Dr given as responsible for certain interventions	`Actor Specification` (e.g. 'Dr') for associated `Role Specification` (e.g. 'responsible for')
Stated: 'This care pathway has been developed by a multidisciplinary team'	`Agent` subtype `Organisation` (i.e. team) who authored the DKA pathway, draft v6
Stated: 'Any comments regarding this care pathway should be directed to Dr X X at site X, ext. xxx'	`Agent` – would be person (the `Care Professional` or [person in] `Role In Organisation`) who is nominated to maintain the care pathway

Explanation: Healthcare professional type viewed separately from the role a person holds within an organisation **Ex**: 'Consultant Diabetologist, Diabetes Specialist Nurse, Staff Nurse'	`Care Professional`
For instance: Carers and patients might contribute to the development of the care pathway, such as advice from their perspective on how information about self-care and prevention of DKA is presented	`Carer(s) and Patient`

Ex:Xxxxxx Acute Hospitals NHS Trust
 	
Ex: The professional role of a clinician within the diabetology unit of the trust. They would be responsible for considering, assigning and ending the care pathway on behalf of a patient, i.e. consultant diabetologist, diabetes specialist nurse, staff nurse, senior staff nurse, ward sister of a particular unit or hospital
	`Organisation`
	
	`Role In Organisation`

Explanation: The care pathway is the chosen means for guiding care and aiding the documentation of clinical information about the patient with DKA	A version of the `Model Care Pathway` is available for use. It spawns a `Care Pathway Use` each time it is used for a patient with DKA
Explanation: Clinical judgement is required for this process, it may be that a care pathway was considered but not used for a patient. This should be recorded. **For instance**: a patient presents in A&E with symptoms of dizziness and thirst. The initial interventions of nil by mouth, urinalysis for general screening, observation and cardiac monitoring (all elements of the DKA care pathway) are engaged, but further assessment indicates the cause of the symptoms to be something else, so the DKA pathway is abandoned.	`Care Pathway Use State` would become 'abandoned'

Continued

Care pathway element from the DKA example . . .	. . . is represented in the model as
Explanation: It is definitely decided to use the Care Pathway for DKA for the patient	Care Pathway Use State **becomes** 'in use'
Explanation: A care pathway can be 'considered', 'in use' where it will be used as a guide for care, or 'ended' for an individual patient. The actual state needs to be identifiable	All would be Care Pathway Use States
Method: The patient sticker that is attached to the care pathway and states name, unit no., D.O.B., sex	Patient
Explanation: The recording of the required information appropriate for the individual patient. **Ex**: known diabetes: Y/N, type: 1,2, insulin-treated type 2, Y/N as to whether obs are recorded with signature and time where appropriate	Patient Characteristic(s) would represent all items of patient history, presentation, observation values, results from screening and test results
Ex: 'patient assessed as confident re urine testing for ketones'. This should be answered after assessing the patient's confidence (an Activity), and where necessary providing training before that (another Activity)	Specific Patient Outcome of related Activity
Encompasses: assessment, monitoring, carrying out tests, making a diagnosis, transferring the patient elsewhere, prescribing, referring, reassessing, educating and supporting the patient, and the recording of these actions. Includes when finished (and when started where duration is significant) AND who played what role in it	Activity and their Activity State(s), Role(s) in Activity (how people participated in the activity) and Actors (who performed those roles)
Method: Interventions done as specified. These are usually indicated with a 'y' as having been done, with a signature by the professional role as indicated and the time where appropriate	Activity As Specified – interventions recorded as having been completed as specified in the Model Care Pathway

Method: Interventions are listed as intended to occur within the first hour, within two hours of admission and within 24 hours; these are recorded, including time, as having been done when expected. The start and finish are given. **Ex**: 6 units/hr of IV continuous variable rate infusion of insulin until capillary blood glucose has fallen to less than 10 mmol/l, then according to sliding scale 1. The actual start, ongoing administration and finish of the 6 units/hr would be recorded on the drugs chart, while a record that this intervention has been prescribed by the doctor is made on the care pathway (this could be done more easily electronically)	Activity State(s) in the Care Pathway Use record when activities were started and finished. When they should have started (and finished, if this is required) is held in the corresponding state change precondition in the Model Care Pathway
Explanation: The clinician who completes or authorises (i.e. prescribes) an intervention for a patient and signs the care pathway accordingly. Also includes the concept of a clinician having the authority to assign a care pathway to a patient in the first place	Role In Activity and who played the role (the Actor)
For instance: If patient was on lithium therapy the Li blood level would need to be known while in an unstable diabetic state	Variance (Patient Characteristic)
For instance: 'N' is ticked for 'technique assessed & educated re insulin therapy' due to patients high anxiety level and fear of needles	Variance – difference between Patient Objective in the Model Care Pathway and the Specific Patient Outcome in the Care Pathway Use
Ex: 'All patients should normally go to HDU or ITU: if patient is transferred to another ward please state where and record reason in multidisciplinary notes'	Modified Activity would represent an activity in the Care Pathway Use that differed from the specification for it in the Model Care Pathway

Continued

Care pathway element from the DKA example . . .	*. . . is represented in the model as*
For instance: taking bloods for Li level would be an additional intervention to the existing care pathway	Extra Activity
For instance: administration of bicarbonate started though the care pathway states that it is rarely recommended. Though initially considered suitable for the patient, it is stopped before completion of course	Ended Activity in the 'abandoned' state
For instance: 'Prophylactic dose of heparin prescribed', but decision is made to not give it due to the patient's other physical problems. No other substitute is prescribed. The intervention is *not required* for this patient **Stated**: 'If an intervention is not carried out for any reason, please tick No and document intervention number, reason and action taken, in multidisciplinary progress notes'	Variant Activity, in this case one that ended in the 'not required' state
For instance: the diabetes specialist nurse is not available to carry out diabetes management teaching for a particular patient, so it is done by the senior staff nurse	**Variance** – the Actor in a Care Pathway Use (who did it) is not the same as the Actor Specification in the Model Care Pathway (who was intended to do it)
Method: Interventions recorded as 'y' with signature. **Ex**: 'Urinalysis for general screening plus ketones recorded', 'date MSU sent' recorded	Activity Completed

Explanation: Consists of the following sub-types or states as it applies to a patient:

1 *Completed* (patient has followed pathway to the end)
   method: Record of discharge – discharge criteria met; date and signature of doctor discharging patient recorded

2 *Discarded* **explanation**: Where the care pathway was considered for a patient, but never actually used. The reason would typically be that the patient's symptoms are not caused by the condition the pathway is designed to treat (in this case DKA)

3 *Abandoned* **explanation**: The pathway is terminated prematurely, because:
   – the patient is transferred to another organisation that does not use this care pathway
   – the patient refuses to continue with care
   – the patient dies

This records how the Care Pathway Use ended. It must be Use Complete, Use Discarded or Use Abandoned. The last two are abnormal end states and include the reason why it was not completed

Ex: The recording that the patient is 'metabolically stable and clinically well, not vomited within 24 hours, eating and drinking, blood sugars less than 20 mmols'

Overall Patient Outcome and Specific Patient Outcome.
The Overall Patient Outcome can be compared with the intended outcome – Overall Objective – in the Model Care Pathway Version. Specific Patient Outcomes – which are specific to an Activity – can be compared with any corresponding Patient Objectives for the corresponding Activity Specification

7

A way forward?

Kathryn de Luc and Julian Todd

Key points

- Embedding evidence-based care pathways in clinical computer systems is a worthwhile goal.

- There is urgent need for a care pathways framework if UK health service targets for computerised care pathways are to be achieved.

- The care pathway framework should consist of the following elements:
  - generic pathways
  - a care pathway community of practice
  - a system for knowledge management and evidence links
  - consistent standards and definitions for care pathways.

Introduction

In the Preface, we described the purpose of the book to be threefold:

- to discuss how one might develop a more systematic approach to care pathway development
- to explore the potential for IT and systems thinking in the further development and implementation of care pathways
- to stimulate debate, discussion and critique about the function and form of e-pathways.

We described the development of care pathways within the UK as 'reinventing wheels on an industrial scale'. We argued that the fragmented approach to their development means that the full potential of care pathways as a quality improvement technique cannot be realised. There are limitations to the concept of care pathways and what they can achieve. Many organisations are facing these limitations on a day-to-day basis. We believe they could be minimised if a different and more structured and systematic approach was taken which utilises the information technology which is available.

We believe that although UK health service policy promotes 'patient-centred' reform and places care pathways firmly within the scope of nationally mandated clinical computer systems, significant progress is not possible using current, conventional approaches.

Summary of the chapters in the book

Chapter 1 described the limitations of current approaches, centred around:

- the need for ongoing clinical evidence management within pathways
- the development, implementation and maintenance of pathways
- the obstacles to moving away from paper-based pathways and embedding them in clinical computer systems
- achieving a whole-community organisational change management approach for care pathways, and finally
- the lack of clarity of the concept and definitions which are universally understood and accepted.

Chapter 2 discussed the importance of assembling and maintaining the knowledge base for care pathways. This is a fundamental requirement if care pathways are to have credibility and fulfil their promise as a vehicle for achieving evidence-based practice. Currently, evidence search activity is almost completely devolved to the individual organisation or health community level. This is a very time- and resource-intensive approach. Multiple evidence citations per care pathway are often held in an *ad hoc* fashion and it is very difficult for users of paper-based care pathways to readily access the evidence for clinical decision support. Maintaining an up-to-date evidence base for clinical practice is a huge task for any clinical member of a multi-professional team, whether they use care pathways or not. The chapter demonstrated an approach to how this could be done within the context of e-pathways.

Chapter 3 concentrated on the development process of care pathways and what is required to manage and support that change. We believe the case study included within this chapter provides a valuable synopsis of the practical issues that can arise when taking different approaches to the development of care pathways. The case study is not enough to draw general conclusions about the pros and cons of the different developmental approaches. However, it can provoke discussion and generate ideas for others to further test the approaches. We think the case study makes a valuable contribution to the debate about the form and feasibility of 'generic' care pathways (see below). This idea rarely gets discussed in the care pathway literature although there are a few projects along similar lines that have been successful. For example, the Welsh Collaborative Care Pathway Project (Fowell *et al.* 2002)[1] had 38 teams introduce the same paper-based care pathway for the dying patient across Wales.

To illustrate how care pathways can be computerised and what is involved in converting a paper-based care pathway to an electronic format, Chapter 4 described one community's experiences. The main lessons from this project are that it is not simply a case of making an electronic version of an already established paper-based care pathway. Instead, the possibilities offered by computerisation require a major rethink and redesign of services. This is a time-consuming task which has to be led by the clinical staff involved.

The second part of this book, which included Chapters 5 and 6, explored how systems approaches could assist with e-pathway development and implementation locally and nationally. Chapter 5 demonstrated the value of applying a systems approach and the accompanying case studies showed how this approach (which is usually the domain of IT or systems specialists) could provide real benefit to clinical staff in their desire to improve services.

Chapter 6 applied similar systems thinking and argued for a national approach to the modelling of the concept of care pathways with the aim of generating debate and discussion so that some nationally accepted standards might emerge. We believe that such national standards are essential for the specification of electronic systems and the computerisation of care pathways. This chapter also briefly reviewed the work via the National electronic Library for Health that is going on to enable the greater accessibility of information and the sharing of care pathways and related information. In our view this facility would benefit organisations immensely and is long overdue.

The argument so far

We believe that the preceding chapters of this book have made the case for the following assertions about care pathways:

- The developing trend towards clinical practice that is evidence based represents an important and permanent shift in clinical professional culture, education and organisation.
- Evidence-based practice is a large and complex knowledge management problem and needs to be managed as such.
- Care pathways are an important quality improvement approach and one of several means of implementing clinical evidence in day-to-day healthcare.
- Care pathways can provide a means for embedding changes in how care is delivered into daily practice. These changes will involve professional roles, cross-agency communications and division of labour etc., focused on the 'patient journey'.
- Care pathways provide a good framework for defining 'clinical workflows', which may include clinical guidelines and protocols.
- Care pathways that are embedded in clinical computer systems have several advantages compared with paper-based pathways (*see* p. 9).
- Structured, systemic change management approaches are required for changes in practice on the scale and at the pace envisaged in UK healthcare policy.

These assertions imply that embedding evidence-based care pathways in clinical computer systems is indeed a valid and worthwhile goal. However, there are problems with the current approach to achieving this. A critical review of current or conventional approaches to care pathway development indicates the following problems:

- Either local health communities are duplicating – wasting – significant effort in developing local pathways from scratch and managing the evidence base locally, or (more often) the overhead of this approach is too great and little or no progress is made.
- The lack of an agreed, explicit structure in paper-based care pathways creates additional work in converting the knowledge they contain into a form suitable for computerisation.
- This lack of structure and standard definitions also limits the ability of communities to share and compare pathways.

Figure 7.1 shows a very broad view of where current approaches to continuous quality improvement, including care pathways, fit into different levels of organisation, i.e. individual patient, clinical team,

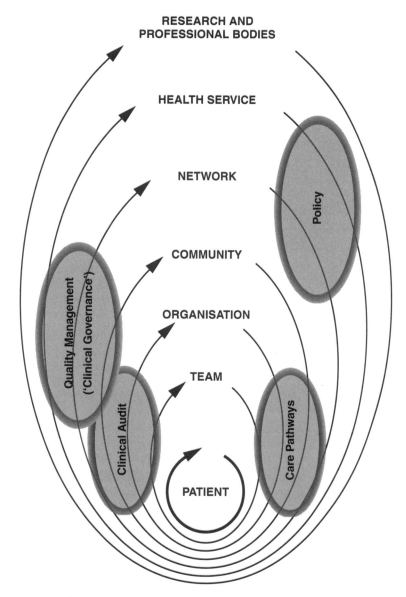

Figure 7.1 Current approaches to continuous quality improvement.

whole organisation, wider community, regional or topic specific networks, health service, and research and professional organisations. The larger arrowed loops indicate both larger-scale undertakings and longer time-scales for change. In the UK, spurred on by some well-publicised whole-systems failures, organisation and community-wide quality management initiatives known as 'clinical governance' have been established. Clinical governance frameworks generally oversee approaches such as clinical audit and care pathways as shown here, together with appraisal, continuing professional development and so on. Policy initiatives are initiated at national level and enacted at whole-organisation level and above, with most of the implementation burden falling on the local organisations.

If e-pathways matter, what might be done to (dis)solve these problems? The rest of this chapter will discuss some developments which we believe may provide some solutions to the problems described.

Proposed developments

Four main developments are described below, which we believe together would form the principal components of a framework for care pathway development and provide a way forward with a reasonable chance of achieving the considerable challenge and opportunity posed by e-pathways.

1 Generic pathways

Further exploration of the concept and practicality of 'generic pathways' is needed. We recognise that this is a contentious and ambitious concept and that further research and discussion is required before the care pathways community would accept it as feasible. Logically, however, if the basic concept of a care pathway as an ideal model of care is valid, then it follows that there must be an underlying similarity of practice across communities and professionals for any given clinical condition.

In developing the concept of generic pathways, we will have to tackle the following issues:

1 Who would authorise the clinical content of the care pathways?
2 Who would authorise best practice in terms of diagnostic and therapeutic interventions to be included in care pathways?
3 How would the form and content of the generic pathway be made independent of local detail?
4 How would the generic pathway be localised and when should it be introduced into the pathway development process?
5 How could we ensure that a sense of local ownership is maintained?

There seems hardly any debate at the moment in the care pathway literature as to the distinctions between generic pathways and valid local pathways. But, in overview, generic pathways would need to:

- reflect roles and functions, not professions or individuals
- be independent of geography and other sources of delay and local variation
- assume optimum availability of skills and resources
- assume optimum work-flow, i.e. be embedded in a scalable model of care which was patient-focused and independent of interfaces between agencies.

Localised pathways, in contrast, would have to reflect local differences in these factors and plan to address any shortfalls compared with the 'optimum'. Example choices/compromises for each aspect outlined above include:

- nurse prescribing and other role variations by grade or profession
- rural versus urban populations and service provision
- the need for professional development in, e.g. new surgical techniques
- funding shortfalls for services locally.

In addition, there would be specific details to be localised such as:

- consensus agreements about treatment where the evidence is not conclusive or where the evidence base was not available
- care pathway cataloguing information
- contact details, department names etc.

Lastly, in order to implement the care pathway in clinical computer systems, the local IT infrastructure and capability would determine which stages or elements of the care pathway would be implemented in which system (across several agencies and organisational boundaries) and which would remain paper based.

A generic care pathway definition would need to be highly structured and contain labels within the structure to identify each element. It would effectively provide a 'skeleton' on which local teams could build. The generic pathway would contain nationally authorised clinical best practice, supported by evidence where available, within a template for clinical work-flow. Local development teams adapting generic pathways should therefore be able to save considerable time and effort at step two (obtaining information on the clinical evidence), step three (scoping the care pathway) and step four (process map and redesign the services) of the ten-step development model outlined in Chapter 1 in Figure 1.1.

2 Community of practice

The idea of a community of practice (CoP) was introduced in Appendix 3.2 of this book. A CoP resource provides an 'on-line' or 'virtual' community of people interested in the topic of (in this instance) care pathways to support more conventional means of education, training and communication. The CoP resource provides e-mail capability, databases, document repositories and on-line discussions or 'computer conferencing', which allow members to add comments to a topic and view others' comments. It has the potential to:

- identify useful initiatives and best practice
- provide a forum for agreeing definitions and standards
- provide a forum for designing and using new national infrastructure to support e-pathways
- support clinical specialist virtual networks to co-operate
- network expertise for moderated evidence and other relevant and related topics.

We appreciate that there have been initiatives to develop this type of approach already,[2-5] but we think that much more could be done to encourage their use at a national/international level. One of the main lessons of trying to set up an electronic network to facilitate care pathway development – previously described in Chapter 3 – is that these virtual communities require time and effort on the part of those setting up the initiative. They do not happen on their own – simply relying on enthusiasts will not be enough.

3 Knowledge management and evidence links in care pathways

The case for a comprehensive and robust knowledge management system based on consistent standards has already been made in Chapter 2.

A system to do this, which is perfectly feasible in IT terms, would include the following:

- A database of evidence moderated by specialists and regularly updated.
- Content which would include summaries, abstracts, references and also full text if copyright was available.
- Evidence cited in generic pathways (and also local ones if agreed by the team) would be linked to the evidence database, so that users of pathways held in a structured electronic format could 'click through' to at least a summary of the supporting evidence. Once implemented in a clinical computer system, this approach would provide much improved decision support capability. A potential international standard to support this approach called Digital Object Identifier system was described in Chapter 2.
- Local communities would register their interest in, or use of, specific generic pathways and therefore be notified by organisations whose role

it is to 'push' information out to the clinicians, e.g. the Virtual Branch Libraries of NeLH (discussed in Chapter 2).
- Organisations could choose to form a mini-CoP, allowing the possibility of 'virtual clinical networks' to co-operate on clinical audit and research projects to more systematically develop evidence where it was lacking. This would allow for immediate access to larger sample sizes to measure the impact of service changes introduced via care pathways.

4 Consistent, structured standards for care pathways

The case for care pathway standards was made in Chapter 6. We believe there needs to be a model which outlines a structure and standards for care pathways. This would contain the 'clinical work-flow' expressed as a hierarchy of stages, steps and tasks, with defined roles, data items and links to other documents. It would also include a definition of software requirements to ensure that suppliers/developers can support e-pathways properly. These standards and structure would be independent of means of implementation, i.e. paper, electronic, work-flow type system, in-house software development and bought-in software.

The purpose would be to:

- support a validation framework to improve care pathway quality
- provide a means of exchanging pathways more easily (e.g. generic to local version, local 1 to local 2 comparison)
- provide a starting point for implementing service redesign (e.g. a template for modernised outpatient services)
- provide a means of more easily implementing care pathways in clinical computer systems
- support the maintenance of the clinical evidence and knowledge management required by care pathways.

To date in the UK, local teams have carried out most of the effort on care pathway development and implementation. At this point in time what is missing is explicit, whole systems management of the topic. What is needed is an overall care pathway framework that involves national and local levels.

An e-pathways framework

The four developments outlined above could provide the principal building blocks of an overall care pathway management framework. Some of the main objectives for this framework are listed below:

- Save time for pathway development teams.
- Improve and validate care pathway quality.
- Maintain relationships between evidence and care pathways over time with minimum effort at local level.
- Provide improved decision support at the patient/clinical professional interface.
- Facilitate networks of clinical specialists and centres of excellence and support the dissemination of expertise throughout the health service.
- Be 'open' and standards based (i.e. non-proprietary).
- Ensure that the structured model for care pathways is as independent as possible from the method of implementation.
- Facilitate diverse approaches to local implementation.
- Provide improved content/document management services for national standard pathways and localised versions.

Figure 7.2 is an updated version of Figure 7.1 showing the four elements of the care pathways framework outlined above. Note that some of the ovals shown on Figure 7.1 are omitted from Figure 7.2 for clarity. The proposed framework is intended to complement and improve existing approaches, not to replace them. A key proposition of the care pathways framework is that a relatively small amount of effort applied at national level would save considerable duplication of effort at local community/organisation/ team level. Thus, generic pathways, standards and knowledge management are all shown facilitated at national level. Knowledge management extends to organisation level, reflecting the need for local clinical library support for care pathway teams in adapting nationally maintained generic pathways and moderated clinical evidence to local circumstances. Care pathways are shown extending beyond the individual team level to whole-community working, which is also the environment for implementation of clinical computing systems. This reflects the aim of integrating services across organisations to support the whole patient journey. We believe that with this kind of framework, the national policy drivers for e-pathways can be realised.

The CoP has the largest extent of all, reflecting the diverse range of individuals and organisations involved in care pathways and related quality improvement and change management initiatives. Some elements of the CoP would be facilitated or managed at national level to support the framework, however spontaneous groupings are likely to emerge 'bottom-up' around either geographic or topic-specific communities. Many examples already exist, but the hope is that the care pathways framework would provide more 'fertile ground' for such groups to grow.

From an information systems perspective, we require a central care pathways catalogue containing an overall model of care, generic

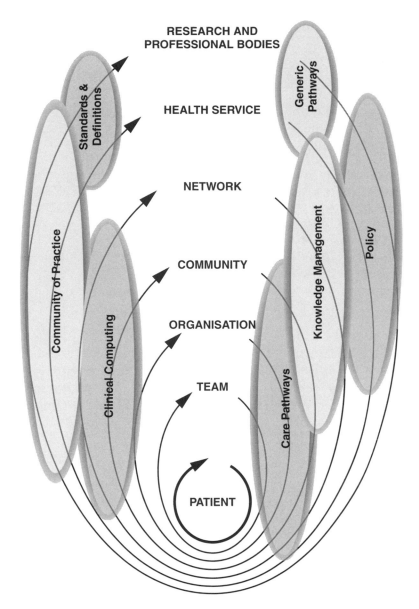

Figure 7.2 e-Pathways framework and continuous quality improvement.

pathways and standard pathway components, linked via citations to a catalogue of moderated evidence. In addition, the IT support system would include:

- a content management system for localised pathways (which could be mirrored at national level to aid co-operation and peer review)
- pathway authoring software for use at national (generic) and local level

- a collaborative framework and on-line community system to support the national CoP and local change management programmes
- a system to alert organisations to changes in generic pathways and moderated evidence base to support the local pathway maintenance effort
- 'how-to' guides on development and implementation of care pathways
- teaching/education on managing change within organisational and professional cultures.

A schematic of the information systems required to support the care pathways framework is shown in Figure 7.3. The four core elements of the framework are shaded, i.e.:

- community of practice
- standards and definitions managed by the NHS Information Authority
- generic care pathways
- knowledge management of the evidence base, which will be moderated as information is fed from local implementation sites applying it.

Figure 7.3 shows how these four components could be applied operationally within the NHS to facilitate local implementation and avoid or reduce the problems identified above. Due to the multi-agency nature of care pathways, all of the elements need to be accessible via the Internet and by non-NHS personnel. We would suggest the NeLH as the national focus, building on what has already been achieved.

Conclusion

This book has highlighted significant weaknesses in the current approach to care pathway development. We have outlined the weaknesses of paper-based care pathways and acknowledged the complexity of change management issues facing any team wishing to develop them. Numerous examples and ideas have been provided as to how information technology and systems-based approaches can help teams and whole communities improve their care pathway work. However, there is a limit to what can be achieved at this level of organisation.

We therefore believe there is an urgent need for a nationally facilitated care pathway management framework if computerised care pathways are going to deliver the benefits expected of them.

We called this book 'e-Pathways' to signify the new approaches we believe are required to development and implementation, if the full potential of computerised care pathways is to be realised with a realistic

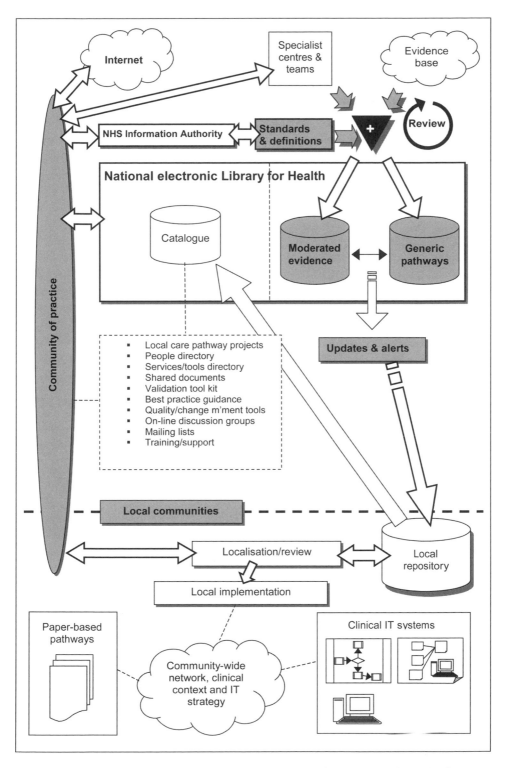

Figure 7.3 Schematic of care pathways framework (shaded).

effort. This book is intended to stimulate and promote an opportunity to debate the future form and function of e-pathways. The ideas contained within this chapter are not a blueprint, but rather a 'thought experiment', a call for a wider debate and, hopefully, concerted action. We hope that if you visit the various sources of further information cited within the book and accompanying CD this process will accelerate.

In Appendix 7.1 we have listed some of the most obvious limitations to the scope of this book and our response. We believe that the limitations identified in fact add further weight to our argument for the greater sharing of ideas and developments about care pathways and e-pathways.

References

1   Fowell A, Finlay I, Johnstone R and Minto L (2002) The Welsh Collaborative Care Pathway Project: implementing an integrated care pathway for the dying patient in Wales. *Journal of Integrated Care Pathways.* **6**: 59–62.
2   http://www.nelh.nhs.uk
3   http://www.smartgroups.com/clinicalpathways
4   http://www.smartgroups.com/groups/care-pathways
5   http://www.venturetc.com/discussion_forum.asp

Appendix 7.1

This appendix summarises the editors' response to the objections which we believe are most likely to be raised as to the purpose and content of the book.

Limitation	Response
The book represents a 'snapshot' of the thinking in 2002 of the various contributors who are working within this field in the UK. We are very aware that there is probably other similar and related work going on around the country and internationally. The problem is that we have no effective way of networking, sharing and learning of similar work and approaches.	The lack of sharing and learning is in itself an argument for the development of the CoP outlined earlier in this chapter as it would encourage other projects to 'make themselves known' and shared. It also provides an opportunity for those with different perspectives (clinical, managerial and IT) to contribute to the debate.
Care pathways are an important quality improvement approach and one of several means of embedding evidence in day-to-day healthcare. Some might argue that the case for care pathways has yet to be proven.[1]	We do not consider it within the remit of this book to summarise the evidence for and against the benefits of introducing care pathways. Our argument about the need for an overall care pathway management framework is in recognition of the complexity of the problem of development and implementation. It is not practicable to set up scientific comparative studies including randomised control trials to measure the impact of e-pathways as we would be trying to measure 'evidence-based social organisation' and there are simply too many variables for this.

Overextension of the care pathway concept. It could be said that many of the limitations of care pathways apply to modern healthcare services in an electronic environment *per se*.

Care pathways are undoubtedly a complex and multifaceted concept – they are much more than simple multidisciplinary records of care or tools to plan healthcare. They embrace both of these ideas and many more, which we believe are central to modern healthcare systems. We believe this provides further weight to our argument for the need for consistent and accepted definitions for the concept of care pathways and associated tools, including guidelines, algorithms and protocols.

[1] Trowbridge R and Weingarten S (2001) *Making Healthcare Safe: a critical analysis of patient safety practices*. Evidence Report/Technology Assessment No. 43. Chapter 52. Prepared for the Agency for Healthcare Research and Quality, www.ahcpr.gov/clinic/ptsafety/chap52.htm.

Care pathway related websites

This section of the book lists over 60 websites which are directly related to care pathways. This list is in addition to the many other sites cited in the various chapters, plus further background material on the CD, although some sites may be listed more than once in different contexts. All web addresses are listed on the CD in a form which should help readers rapidly select and access sites which are relevant to their needs.

The list has been compiled with the help of Alan Fisher, Ross Scrivener and Kris Vanhaecht, as noted in the Preface. At the time of writing we hope that the list and other resources collected during the production of the book will be added to the care pathway information already available on-line via the NeLH. Your attention is drawn in particular to the NeLH website http://www.nelh.nhs.uk. This site includes a care pathway database containing citations and contact details for over 2000 pathways, plus full text of 100 sample pathways, and there are plans to further extend the information available on this site in the near future.

The editors have made all reasonable efforts to check that website addresses and hyperlinks are accurate and up to date, however this cannot be guaranteed. A more up to date version of the website list can be found on the CD. This is not intended to be an exhaustive list of care pathway sites and inclusion of a site in the list does not imply that the editors endorse or promote the content.

The list is divided into the following sections:

- General information
- Bibliographical lists
- On-line literature
- Examples of care pathways
- Supporting organisations
- Projects
- IT support.

Website address	Bookmark entry	Description
General information on care pathways		
http://www.ahca.org/news/provider/pv9808cg.htm	American Health Care Association	Organisation: American Health Care Association – the association of long-term care in the community
http://www.consorta.com/wings/depts/oe/clin_path/	Consorta Catholic Resource Partners	Sample pathways, how to develop + template. Organisation: Consorta Catholic Resource Partners
http://dva.gov.au/health/provider/community%20nursing/pathways/pathindex.htm	Dept. of Veterans' Affairs	Sample guidelines and care pathways. Organisation: Department of Veterans' Affairs, Australia
http://www.evidence-based-medicine.co.uk/ebmfiles/whatisanicp.pdf	Evidence-based medicine	Published by Hayward Medical Communications
http://www.hsurc.sk.ca/resource_centre/care/index.php3	Health Services Utilization and Research Commission	Getting-started guide. Organisation: Health Services Utilization and Research Commission
http://www.ipswichhospital.org.uk/icp/icpmain.htm	Ipswich Hospital NHS Trust	Includes sample pathways and general description. Organisation: Ipswich Hospital NHS Trust

http://www.multiplan.com/providers/libraryservices/?libraryid=1	Library of critical paths – Multiplan	Holds library of critical paths. To gain access must join Multiplan's nationwide (USA) healthcare network and contribute own pathways. Organisation: Multiplan
http://ifmss.org.uk/publics/msmgmt/sept95/icp.htm	Care pathways & multiple sclerosis	Information relating specifically to care pathways and multiple sclerosis. Organisation: Multiple Sclerosis International Federation
http://pedsccm.wustl.edu/CLINICAL/Pathways.html	Critically ill infants & children	Sample pathways, references etc. All relate to critically ill infants and children. Organisation: PedsCCM: clinical pathways and guidelines
http://wwwsvh.stvincents.com.au/qi/Clin_Pathways	St Vincent's Hospital	Bibliographic list – under useful clinical pathway resources. Sample pathways. Organisation: St Vincent's Hospital, Sydney
http://www.bmido.com/pathway.htm	Taiwan	General information and sample pathways from Taiwan
http://www.system.missouri.edu/hrs/comp/spec2/2814.htm	Job description – pathway co-ordinator	Job description for clinical pathways outcomes co-ordinator. Organisation: University of Missouri System

Continued

Website address	Bookmark entry	Description
http://www.health.vic.gov.au http://aca.health.vic.gov.au/critpath.htm	Victorian Govt. Health Info	Various information on both sites, includes evaluation framework for care pathways. Organisation: Victorian Government Health Information Ambulatory Care, Australia
http://www.asahq.org/NEWSLETTERS/1998/10_98/ Why_1098.html	Pathway implementation citations	Article on evidence base for pathways as quality and cost control tool. Organisation: American Society of Anesthesiologists

Bibliographical lists on care pathways

Website address	Bookmark entry	Description
http://www.aapmr.org	American Academy of Physical Medicine & Rehab	Bibliographic list specifically for physical medicine and rehabilitation clinical pathways. Organisation: American Academy of Physical Medicine and Rehabilitation
http://www.the-npa.org	National Pathways Association	Bibliographic list available to non-members. Organisation: National Pathways Association

http://pedscccm.wustl.edu/CLINICAL/Pathways.html	Infants & children	References, general information, sample pathways etc. All relate to critically ill infants and children. Organisation: PedsCCM: clinical pathways and guidelines
http://www.springnet.com	Springnet	Search for clinical paths etc. and various references listed. Organisation: Springnet – on-line nursing information
http://wwwsvh.stvincents.com.au/qi/Clin_Pathways	St Vincent's	Bibliographic list – under useful clinical pathway resources. Sample pathways. Organisation: St Vincent's Hospital, Sydney
http://www.nlm.nih.gov/pubs/cbm/critpath.html	US Nat. Lib. of Medicine	Bibliographic list 1988–1995. Organisation: United States National Library of Medicine
http://www.cmaj.ca	Canadian Medical Association Journal	Searchable database of articles and pathways, including full text. Organisation: Canadian Medical Association
http://mayday.coh.org	City of Hope	Palliative care/pain relief resources, including pathways. Organisation: City of Hope Pain/ Palliative Care Resource Centre & Beckman Institute

Continued

On-line literature about care pathways

Website address	Bookmark entry	Description
http://www.allenpress.com/searchframes.html	Article on older patients	Assessing the efficacy of a clinical pathway in the management of older patients. Organisation: Allen Press
http://www.acponline.org/journals/ecp/mayjun02/darer.pdf	Article on eval. of pathways in hospitals	Use and evaluation of critical pathways in hospitals. Organisation: ACP-ASIM on-line (American College of Physicians and American Society of Internal Medicine)
http://www.ahcpr.gov/clinic/ptsafety/chap52.htm	Report on eval. of pathways AHRQ	*Making Healthcare Safer: a critical analysis of patient safety practices*. Evidence Report/Technology Assessment No. 48. Chapter 52. Organisation: Agency for Healthcare Research and Quality
http://www.jr2.ox.ac.uk/bandolier/band101/b101-2.html#heading 3../index.html	Article on eval. of pathways Bandolier	Review of the research studies measuring the effectiveness of care pathways. Organisation: Bandolier

URL	Description	Details
http://www.bmj.com/misc/qhc/30-36.shtml	Article mapping out the patient's journey	Mapping out the patient's journey: experiences of developing pathways of care. Can search site for other citations. Organisation: British Medical Journal
http://www.mja.com.au/public/issues/jan18/dowsey/dowsey.html	Article on pathways in hip & knee arthroplasty	Clinical pathways in hip and knee arthroplasty: a prospective randomised controlled study. Can search for other citations. Organisation: EMJA The Medical Journal of Australia
http://www.dis.port.ac.uk/~norrist/shimr99js.html	Paper on pathways & info for health	*Care Pathways and the Information for Health Strategy* policy document. Authors: Norris AC and Briggs JS. Organisation: Portsmouth University

Examples of care pathways

URL	Description	Details
http://www.nelh.nhs.uk	Care pathway database	Care pathway database – UK wide. Organisation: National electronic Library for Health

Continued

Website address	Bookmark entry	Description
http://pedsccm.wustl.edu/CLINICAL/Pathways.html	Critically ill infants & children	Sample pathways, references, general information etc. All relate to children. Organisation: PedsCCM: clinical pathways and guidelines
http://wwwsvh.stvincents.com.au/qi/Clin_Pathways	St Vincent's examples	Sample pathways, general information, bibliographic list – under useful clinical pathway resources. Organisation: St Vincent's Hospital, Sydney
http://www.bmido.com/pathway.htm	Taiwan examples	Sample pathways and general information
http://www.uq.edu.au/cgpmh/gp-paths/gp-00intro.htm	Mater Mothers examples	Antenatal, postnatal and diabetic pathways for combined primary/ secondary care. Organisation: Mater Mothers Hospital, Queensland, Australia
http://www.medschl.cam.ac.uk/phgu/info_database/ care_pathways/care_pathways.asp	Scottish Genetics examples	Pathways on tuberous sclerosis (TS), myotonic dystrophy (MD), Marfan syndrome, Huntington's disease (HD) and Neurofibromatosis 1 (NF1). Organisation: Scottish Clinical Genetics Service

URL	Name	Description
http://www.dva.gov.au/health/provider/community%20nursing/pathways/woundmgt.htm http://www.dva.gov.au/health/provider/community%20nursing/pathways/respire.htm	Veterans' Affairs examples	Wound management and respiratory pathways. Organisation: Department of Veterans' Affairs, Australia

Supporting organisations/networks/discussion forums and consultants

URL	Name	Description
http://www.nkp.be	Belgian CP Network – NKP	Network of 30 hospitals working together on clinical pathways and co-ordinated by the Centre for Health Services and Nursing Research, Catholic University, Leuven, Belgium. Organisation: Belgium–Dutch Clinical Pathway Network
http://www.robertluttman.com/Week6/index.htm http://www.robertluttman.com/monograph.html	Luttman	Provides an educational seminar on pathways and general support. Organisation: Bob Luttman, Robert Luttman & Associates
http://www.icpus.ukprofessionals.com	Scottish CP Network	General information about network in Scotland. Organisation: Integrated Care Pathway Users Scotland

Continued

Website address	Bookmark entry	Description
http://www.the-npa.org	National Pathways Association	Have to be a member of organisation to gain access to the discussion forum. Organisation: National Pathways Association
http://www.cfcm.com	Centre for Case Management	Healthcare consultancy company. Includes: specific products, seminars, publications, information on clinical path automation. Organisation: Centre for Case Management
http://www.smartgroups.com/groups/carepathways	Smart Group – MH	Discussion forum: mental health focus
http://www.smartgroups.com/clinicalpathways	Smart Group – General	Discussion forum for care pathways
http://www.venturetc.co.uk	Venture Consulting	Healthcare consultancy company. Includes: training courses, support and discussion forums. Organisation: Venture Training and Consulting

http://www.nelh.nhs.uk/heart/racpcs/dataset/index.htm	RACPC	Rapid Access Chest Pain Clinic (RACPC) project. Includes generic specification for RACPC information system, chest pain flow-chart, patient information and decision support/advice. Organisation: National electronic Library for Health
http://www.curapath.com/webpages/news.html	Northampton projects	Information about specific care pathway project. Organisation: Northampton General Hospital + Curapath
http://www.icpathways.org.uk	N. & Yorks. projects	Information about an action learning programme on care pathways. Organisation: NHS Executive Northern & Yorkshire Region Funded Collaborative Project between the University of Teeside School of Health, York Department of Health and Economics and South Tees Acute NHS Trusts
http://www.orthopaedic.ed.ac.uk/research.htm	Orthopaedic projects	Information about specific research project on elective orthopaedic pathways. Organisation: Princess Margaret Rose Orthopaedic Hospital, Edinburgh

Continued

Website address	Bookmark entry	Description
http://www.nyx.org.uk/modernprogrammes/patientaccess/goodpractice/feb2002/pathway.html	Hartlepool projects	Hartlepool General Hospital – progress with implementation. Organisation: The Northern and Yorkshire Regional NHS Modernisation Programme
http://dialspace.dial.pipex.com/town/estate/xap45/f5.htm	Dorset Osteoporosis project	Information about specific project in care pathways and osteoporosis. Organisation: Osteoporosis Dorset
http://www.shef.ac.uk/~scharr/publich/research/carepath.html	Sheffield Cardiovascular project	Information about specific project on cardiovascular disease care pathways. Organisation: University of Sheffield

IT support

Website address	Bookmark entry	Description
www.qmedit.be	Qmedit Software	Software for pathway development, deployment and variance analysis
http://www.zynx.com/Products/products-cpc.htm	Clinical Pathway Constructor	Pathway and guideline builder and database
http://www.thornberryltd.com	NDoc Software	Clinical documentation builder
http://www.excelcare.com/clinicalpaths.htm	EXCELCARE software	Care planning and documentation system

http://www.qworks.com/	Q-Works software	Clinical quality management software for pathway development, deployment and variance analysis
http://www.curapath.com/	Curapath software	Software for pathway development, deployment and variance analysis
http://www.achievehealthcare.com/pltour/pltour.htm	Pathlinks software	Clinical process management – financial focus
http://www.ergopartners.com/ErgoWeb1V2_3.htm	EMRitus software	Protocol and disease management software
http://www.clinicomp.com/products-clinicalpath.html	Clinical Pathway Administrator	Care pathway module of Clinicomp International clinical computing system

See also Appendix B of report cited in the Introduction (*see* p. 3) for additional IT-related sites: Flower J, Geernaert M and Hartshorn A (2001) *Review of Issues and Options for Creating, Storing and Using Electronic Care Pathways across the NHS.* BBD Consultancy Services, Lichfield. Full text on CD.

Glossary

The following brief definitions of terms and acronyms used in the book are provided to help readers who are not specialists in information technology and/or who are not familiar with the UK health service. Clinical examples are used where possible. Text shown in **bold** in a definition is a cross-reference to another definition.

Active Server Pages (ASP)	Technique for dynamically creating pages of information on the **World Wide Web** from a **database**. **Web** pages created from a **database** automatically display changes to the **data**, as opposed to static web pages, which have to be manually updated.
Attribute	Detailed part of the definition of a **class** in **UML**.
Booking	Term used within the **NHS** for a development programme designed to offer greater choice to patients in the time and place of their appointment, such as a specialist consultant clinic or day-case surgery. The most recent development in the programme is 'e-booking' which allows appointments to be automatically booked via a computer screen (as opposed to a letter or phone call).
Browser	Shorthand term for the type of **software** required to access the **World Wide Web**, as in the expression 'point your browser at the **NeLH** website'.
Business rule	Term used in design of computer systems and **databases**, meaning an unambiguous, detailed course of action which must be followed when certain conditions are met. *See* **Rules**.

Care pathway	Several definitions are offered in this book, all of which emphasise that care pathways are both an ideal model of care for a given condition and a way of recording relevant details of what actually happened during the care of a specific individual. Usually care pathways are developed and used by many professions and agencies to reflect the whole 'patient journey' through the healthcare system.
Change management	Systematic approach to the management of large-scale change in complex organisations.
Class	Within a **software** modelling language such as **UML**, a detailed description of a set of objects which share attributes, behaviour and relationships (with other classes).
Community	*See* **Health community**.
Computerisation	Conversion of work activities from paper-based or 'manual' format to computer software. Thus, paper forms would be converted to forms on computer screens; the ways in which the forms are processed and filed would be converted into software rules, with a database to store the data on the form.
Configuration	Detailed set-up and reference files needed to make computer **software** work in specific circumstances. For example, the word processor such as that used to write this book has country setting (= UK), grammar checking function (= off) etc.
CoP	Community of Practice. Term within the field of **Knowledge management**, for a group with a common interest organised in a way that encourages sharing of information and skills.
Data	Elemental item operated on by a computer; quantity (of something). Digital computers operate on data coded as binary numbers, i.e. zero or one are the only allowable states, known as a 'bits' (**b**inary di**g**its). Computer data is commonly stored and operated on in multiples of 'bytes' – where a byte is eight bits. Volumes of data are measured in bytes – the character 'a' is stored as two bytes (16 bits) in a modern personal computer. Whole files of data typically occupy many kilobytes (Kb),

megabytes (Mb) or even gigabytes (Gb) for large, high-definition digital images. These units represent respectively approximately 1000 bytes, 1 000 000 bytes and 1 000 000 000 bytes.

Database
Term for both a structured collection of **data** and the **software** required to manage the data.

Data set
Collection of **data** applying to a specific context, e.g. Lung Cancer Clinical Data Set, which includes data items describing attributes of the patient, tumour, treatments etc.

Decision support
General term for the provision of detailed information in a specific context where a specialist has to make a key decision. The term originated in management information systems, but in a clinical computer system it would include any information to support accurate diagnosis and assessment of treatment options, e.g. access to information on drug interactions.

Decision tree
Logical sequence of conditions or tests which have multiple branches and ultimately outcomes from the whole tree. These are often presented as a **flow chart** or similar diagram.

Digital Object Identifier (DOI)
Technique for uniquely referencing and accessing 'units of information' – articles, books, pictures etc. via the **Internet**.

Domain name
Equivalent of an address of a service on the **Internet**, expressed in a way which can be understood by people, whereas computers store their addresses as numbers. Domains are hierarchical and domain names are read from left to right, lowest level to highest level. Levels are separated by the full stop character '.', pronounced 'dot'. Thus '.com' (commonly known as 'dot com') is the commerce domain; '.gov' is the government domain and so on. Thus in the web address 'http://www.nlm.nih.gov/mesh', the domain name is 'nlm.nih.gov' (National Library of Medicine, which is part of the National Institute for Health, which is part of the [US] government). Domain names must be unique and therefore have to be registered on the **Internet**.

Download	Act of copying information from one computer (usually the larger one) to another, via some form of data communications system.
Electronic health record (EHR)	Concept within the UK **NHS** framework for clinical information systems, which is a summary record of conditions and treatments for a specific patient during their lifetime, plus key clinical data such as blood group, allergies etc.
Electronic patient record (system) (EPR)	UK **NHS** framework for clinical information systems. Defined in levels from 1 to 6, where level 6 is a fully electronic clinical system. Level 3 is a national target for all acute hospitals, which includes the capability to support computerised care pathways.
Elementary business process (EBP)	Term used in formal **process** analysis to describe a 'unit of work' which is carried out by one person (or small team) at one time and place to achieve a specific goal. An EBP usually comprises several **tasks**.
e-pathway	General term used throughout the book to summarise the application of information technology to care pathway development and implementation. Compare with 'e-mail', 'e-commerce', 'e-government'.
Fishbone diagram	Type of diagram (also known as an Ishikawa diagram or Cause & Effect diagram) which supports small-group discussion and agreement about a topic or problem. The name originated because the diagram resembles a side-on view of a fish skeleton.
Flow chart	Originally, a type of diagram used in designing the detailed logic of computer software. Flow charts have fallen out of use in **IT**, but they are often now used to model sets of logical decisions, such as triage.
Generic pathway	Definition of a care pathway, which identifies best evidence for a specific clinical condition and the main steps and tasks to achieve a clinical goal, but which is independent of local implementation details.

Guideline

Evidence-based, detailed description of the treatment recommended for a specific condition or set of symptoms, usually for use by a single profession.

Hardware

Physical electronics and equipment in a computer which process the instructions contained in **software**. Hardware is often subdivided into modules for **data** input, processing, storage and output.

Health community

Set of organisations and professions which provide and manage health and social care in a geographic area. In the UK, there would be a mix of publicly-funded, local government, private sector and voluntary organisations, although the largest proportion of care would be delivered by the **NHS**.

Human–computer interface (HCI)

General term for the way in which people interact with computers. Related terms include 'graphical user interface (GUI)', '**browser** (or **web**) interface', 'windows interface', which all refer to similar styles of HCI. The common elements are movable frames (windows) for information display, a computer mouse and on-screen pointer to select items on the screen, and icons – illustrated buttons – which can be selected to perform software functions.

Hyperlink

Highlighted word, phrase or icon embedded in text displayed on a computer screen, which allows the user to jump directly to another section or file of information. See **hypertext**.

Hypertext

Way of presenting and managing information (usually text and diagrams) on a computer which allows the reader to jump directly from one section to another via **hyperlinks**. The concept and first working examples were developed in the 1970s, but this approach to presenting information has only become commonplace with the emergence of the **World Wide Web**. *See also* **HTML**.

HyperText Mark-up Language (HTML)

Set of standard codes which are embedded in computer files to specify how the information is to be displayed on-screen by web browser software. The codes are not displayed. A key element of **HTML** is the use of **hyperlinks** to allow users to jump almost instantaneously to related information elsewhere on the **Internet**. **HTML** is the basis of the **World Wide Web**.

Informatics	Broad term for the scientific study and application of information and **IT**, in the same sense that 'electronics' covers the field of the science and technology of electricity.
Information	Items of knowledge. Data becomes information when it is put into a human context. It is often placed in a hierarchy thus: data; information; knowledge (how to apply information). Wisdom, as the accumulated experience of knowing when or how to apply knowledge to good effect, is perhaps best considered separately.
Information and communications technology (ICT)	More recent term than **IT**, highlighting the process of convergence between IT and data communications, for example use of mobile phones to send and receive electronic mail and access the Internet. The term 'information management and technology' (IM&T) is also used in the **NHS** to include the area of provision of information for health service management.
Information technology (IT)	Broad term covering the practical details of computing and its application to practical situations.
Integrated Care Record System (ICRS)	Most recent **NHS** specification (c.2002) for clinical computing systems.
Internet	Global network linking millions of separate computer systems, which provides several types of information service. The most well known service is the **World Wide Web** (WWW).
Intranet	Information service using **Internet** technical standards, but available only to people within one organisation or community.
Knowledge management (KM)	Broad term for the systematic study and management of how knowledge is created, used, communicated and recorded, usually within one (large) organisation or subject area. Related terms are 'knowledge worker', 'knowledge capital',

'knowledge economy', which all reflect the fact that in the developed world at least, the economy is evolving away from a manufacturing base towards the production and processing of knowledge in all its forms.

Medical subject headings (MeSH)	Set of several hundred thousand clinical terms and associated codes, which provide a standard clinical taxonomy. This is commonly used to catalogue and search for citations in the medical literature. MeSH is stronger in medical areas and has a USA cultural bias.
Menu	List of optional actions within a computer program, displayed as a list to the user.
Messaging	Verb and noun describing a particular way of linking different computers through exchange of structured messages (each of which would contain an agreed data set). For example, a discharge summary following a patient stay in an acute hospital could be sent as a message to the computer system of the patient's general practitioner. General-purpose electronic mail systems are commonly used to transport such messages.
Methodology	Explicitly defined way of tackling a particular problem or set of problems. For example, PRojects IN a Controlled Environment (PRINCE) is a project management methodology; Structured Systems Analysis and Design Methodology (SSADM) is a computer software development methodology – both of these are UK government sponsored.
Mind map	Type of diagram devised by Tony Buzan in the 1960s, which allows an individual or small group to rapidly note down and structure issues and ideas related to a central topic. Mind maps are superior to simple lists because they encourage creative thinking about the whole topic and can grow organically.
Multimedia	Term for the application of computing to graphic art and presentation of information using combinations of text, sound, pictures and video, usually

	within a structure which allows the viewer to move through the presentation at their own pace. Modern web browser software is capable of handling multimedia.
National electronic Library for Health (NeLH)	Main health information site in the UK.
National Health Service (NHS)	Main organisation providing healthcare in the UK, which is funded through taxation and is generally free to use. There are variations in how the service is managed between England, Wales, Scotland and Northern Ireland.
NHS Information Authority (NHSIA)	National agency responsible for developing and managing IT infrastructure and technical standards: www.nhsia.nhs.uk.
NHS Information Policy Unit (IPU)	Part of the central **NHS** management structure responsible for policy and strategy.
On-line	State of being connected to a remote computer via a data communications system. It is also used in expressions such as 'on-line community', meaning a group of people with a common interest or purpose who communicate mainly via computers.
Procedure	General term for a specific clinical/therapeutic intervention, e.g. tonsillectomy.
Process	Set of related activities to achieve a goal. Since process analysis is recursive, the same term may apply to a very abstract, high-level description or a much more detailed description of the activities. See also **EBP**.
Process chart	Low-level view of a **process** comprising **elementary business processes** and their interrelationships.
Process map	High-level view of an overall **process** showing the main subprocesses and their interrelationships.
Protocol	Detailed set of actions and forms designed to handle a specific healthcare problem, usually representing a mandatory joint agreement between professions or agencies, for example a referral protocol from a general practitioner to a specialist consultant for patients with suspected breast cancer.

Rules | In the context of this book, a clinical rule such as 'change fluid type to 10% glucose when capillary blood glucose has fallen to less than 10 mmol per litre'. *See* **business rule**.

Security model | General term for the way in which user access to a computer system containing confidential information is managed. A security model would include policies and procedures; methods for connecting and disconnecting to the system (known respectively as logging in and logging out); rules stating which types of user could view and change which parts of the **data set** or authorise actions and messages; ways of monitoring user actions. Example: 'Only consultant grade doctors can authorise requests for blood products and all such requests will be recorded.'

Software | Broad term for the set of instructions which make a general-purpose computer perform useful functions. The counterpart to **hardware**. The word is often preceded by a qualifier indicating the type of function, e.g. word-processing software, database software. Note also the growing list of derivative terms such as 'vapourware' (software which is promised, but not delivered). A common synonym of 'software' is '(computer) program'.

Symbolic modelling | Structured framework for modelling complex systems where the objects in the model and their interrelationships are defined and stored in a **database**. Definitions can be associated with symbols, which can be placed on diagrams, which are also stored in the database.

Systemic | In systems thinking, an approach which addresses the 'whole system', i.e. which is not reductionist and which assumes that the 'whole is greater than the sum of its parts'.

System-in-focus | Term used in systems analysis to refer to the main system being modelled. Since systems thinking is recursive, it is possible in principle to break down any system into many levels of sub-systems. In practice this is rarely helpful; usually a maximum of three system levels is sufficient.

Tasks — Elemental action within an **elementary business process**, for example 'insert cannula'; 'request full blood count'.

Trust — In the UK **NHS**, the legal framework for those organisations in the service which provide clinical care.

Unified Modelling Language (UML) — International standard method for specifying **software**.

Universal Resource Locator — Technical term within the HyperText Transfer Protocol for the address of a website. It is commonly known as a 'web address'. *See* **World Wide Web**.

User interface — *See* **Human–computer interface** (HCI).

Web — Short for **World Wide Web**, as in 'web address', 'website', 'web browser'.

Work-flow — Similar to process, but more specifically to do with the organisation of human labour, especially a sequence of actions, authorisations and transfers of objects and information between people to achieve a shared goal.

World Wide Web (WWW) — Collective name for all the computers on the **Internet** which use a particular type of **hypertext** information service, devised by Tim Berners-Lee in the early 1980s to improve communications between scientific research communities around the world. WWW allows a 'web' of linked information pages to be created and is much easier to create and use than previous generations of Internet information-sharing services. Access to web pages requires a specialised software package called a web **browser**. Examples include *Mosaic*, *Microsoft Internet Explorer* and *Netscape Navigator*. The hypertext service is known as HyperText Transfer Protocol (HTTP), which is why the full specification of a website is written (for example) http://www.nelh.nhs.uk.

Index

access arrangements, health knowledge
31–2
assertions, care pathways 186–8
assistance sources, care pathways 63–6,
76–80
Athens Authentication Service 32
audit and feedback, care pathway
development 57

barriers
communication 58–9
evidence-based practice 94–7
behaviour, facilitation 64–5
best practices, healthcare map 21–4
bibliographic databases 40
BPR *see* business process re-engineering
Brown, SJ 21–4
business process re-engineering (BPR)
117–18

Care Pathway Conceptual Structure 159,
160–72
concepts, main 160–3
developing 160
DKA 166–71, 174–81
example 166–71
overview 163–6
care pathways
approaches 69–75
assertions 186–8
assistance sources 63–6, 76–80
benefits 2–3
case studies 47–50, 69–75, 83

change agenda 46–7
change management approach 10
change, managing 50
concept map ix
consensus building 59–60
consistency/inconsistency 10–12
coronary heart disease 48
defining 1–3, 139, 158
development 5–7, 19–21, 46–80, 72–3
developments, proposed 188–91
ethos 1–3
evidence-based practice 4–5
facilitation 62–3, 64–5
implementation 5–7, 73–5
implementation strategies 53–4
leadership 60–1
learning disabilities 47–8
limitations 3–12
maintenance 5–7
modelling approach 110–13, 114–17
negotiation 59–60
paper-based 7–10, 89, 91–3
people, influencing 51–2
planning 69–72
process maps 29, 129–31, 140–2, 149–51
process redesign 117–18
resistance, dealing with 54–9
stroke services 48–9
Systems Architect example 149–54
systems perspective 113–14
systems view 109–54
teamworking 52–3
websites 35–9, 199–211
see also computerised care pathways

case studies
  care pathways 47–50, 69–75
  chest pain 28–31
  computerised care pathways 83
  flow charts 129–31
  FlowForma 128
  knowledge management 28–31
  myocardial infarction 28–31
  process maps 129–31
  SSM 121–6
  stroke services 121–6
  systems view 120–31
  TOC 127
change
  Dudley change programme 132–42
  managing 50, 118–20
  whole-organisation level 118–20
change agenda, care pathways 46–7
change management approach, care
    pathways 10
chest pain, case study 28–31
CINAHL see Cumulative Index to Nursing
    and Allied Health Literature
clinical audit, cyclical change
    management 118–20
clinical guidelines
  appraisal tools 37
  defining 157
  knowledge management 24–5
  MEDLINE 24–5
  websites 37
clinical protocol, defining 157
clinical trials, websites 38
Cochrane Effective Practice and
    Organisation of Care (EPOC) 54, 55–7
communication
  barriers 58–9
  framework, Dudley change programme
    135
  and involvement 58
Community of Practice (CoP) 79–80
  developments, proposed 189–90, 191–4
computed tomography (CT) 116
computer software see software
computer-supported cooperative work
    (CSCW) 78–9
computerised care pathways 81–108
  background 82
  case study 83
  construction 85–94
  development time 93–4

IT requirement 86–7
  lessons learnt 94–7
  rules 93
  scope 87–91
  screen shots examples 99–105
  stroke services 83–108
  tasks 93
  transitions 94–7
  see also care pathways
conferences, care pathway development
    55
consensus building, care pathways 59–60
consensus process, care pathway
    development 55
consistency/inconsistency, care pathways
    10–12
continuous quality improvement 186–8,
    192–3
CoP see Community of Practice
coronary heart disease, care pathways 48
critical appraisal, evidence 25–6
CSCW see computer-supported
    cooperative work
CT see computed tomography
Cumulative Index to Nursing and Allied
    Health Literature (CINAHL) 139

development, care pathways 5–7, 19–21,
    46–80, 72–3
developments, proposed 188–91
diabetic ketoacidosis (DKA) 142, 145–8,
    149–54
  Care Pathway Conceptual Structure
    166–71, 174–81
Digital Object Identifier (DOI) 32
DILEMMA initiative 159
directive facilitation 65
DKA see diabetic ketoacidosis
DOI see Digital Object Identifier
drug information, websites 38
Dudley change programme 132–42

education, websites 39
educational materials, care pathway
    development 55
educational outreach visits, care pathway
    development 56
EHRs see electronic health records
electronic health records (EHRs) 82
Electronic Patient Records (EPRs) 138,
    140

Electronic Record Development and
    Implementation Programme (ERDIP)
    172
EPOC *see* Cochrane Effective Practice and
    Organisation of Care
EPRs *see* Electronic Patient Records
ERDIP *see* Electronic Record Development
    and Implementation Programme
ethos, care pathways 1–3
evaluation *see* critical appraisal, evidence
evidence base effectiveness,
    implementation strategies 55–7
evidence-based practice
    barriers 94–7
    care pathways 4–5
evidence, critical appraisal, knowledge
    management 25–6

facilitation
    behaviour 64–5
    care pathways 62–3, 64–5
feedback and audit, care pathway
    development 57
flow charts, case study 129–31
FlowForma, case study 128
follow-up, stroke services 88–93
framework, e-pathways 191–4, 195

generic pathways, developments,
    proposed 188–9, 191–4
glossary 213–22
guidelines, clinical *see* clinical guidelines

health knowledge, access arrangements
    31–2
healthcare map, best practices 21–4
Heart Diseases Virtual Branch Library
    28–31

implementation
    care pathways 73–5
    strategies 53–4, 55–7
influencing people 51–2
information
    NHSIA 156
    patient 39
Information for Health 133, 156
information needs, identifying, knowledge
    management 19–21
information searching protocols,
    knowledge management 21–4

Internet
    knowledge management 35–9
    search engines 42
    search tools 43
    surfing reasons 35–9
involvement, and communication 58

knowledge management 17–43
    access arrangements, health knowledge
        31–2
    case study 28–31
    clinical guidelines 24–5
    developments, proposed 190–1, 191–4
    evidence, critical appraisal 25–6
    information needs, identifying 19–21
    information searching protocols 21–4
    librarians, healthcare 18–19
    resource discovery tools 40–3
    updating knowledge base 26–7

leadership, care pathways 60–1
learning disabilities, care pathways 47–8
librarians, healthcare, knowledge
    management 18–19

managing change 50, 118–20
marketing, care pathway development 57
Medical Subject Headings (MeSH) 139
MEDLINE, clinical guidelines 24–5
MeSH *see* Medical Subject Headings
modelling approach
    care pathways 110–13, 114–17
    characteristics, good models 114–15
    Dudley change programme 132–42
    software 133–42
    standards 156–8, 159–60
    stroke services 125
    symbolic modelling 138
    Systems Architect 133–42
    whole-organisation level 118–20
Modernisation Agency 63–6
multifaceted interventions, care pathway
    development 57
myocardial infarction, case study 28–31

National electronic Library for Health
    (NeLH) 171–2
National Pathways Association (NPA)
    158–9
negotiation, care pathways 59–60
NeLH *see* National electronic Library for
    Health

news, websites 39
NHS Information Authority (NHSIA) 156, 171–2
The NHS Plan 112
NPA *see* National Pathways Association

objections responses 197–8
official information, websites 38–9
opinion leaders, care pathway development 56
Ovid 27

paper-based care pathways 7–10, 89, 91–3
patient information, websites 39
patient-mediated interventions, care pathway development 56
people, influencing 51–2
personality approaches 51–2
persuasive facilitation 64
planning, care pathways 69–72
PRESTIGE initiative 159
primary research
    digest 35–7
    reviews 35
    websites 38
process maps
    care pathways 29, 140–2, 149–51
    case study 129–31
    DKA 149–51
process redesign, care pathways 117–18
PubMed 27
purpose, this book's viii, 183

quality, continuous quality improvement 186–8

reasons
    Internet surfing 35–9
    for this book vi–viii
reductionist approach, cf. systemic approach 110–13, 115
reminders, care pathway development 57
research, primary *see* primary research
resistance, dealing 54–9
resource discovery tools 40–3
reviews, primary research 35

screen shots examples, computerised care pathways 99–105
soft systems methodology (SSM) 115–16
    case study 121–6

software
    assistance sources 76–80
    benefits 134–5, 136
    comparison 137
    modelling approach 133–42
    Systems Architect 133–42, 149–54
SSM *see* soft systems methodology
standards
    developing 155–81
    developments, proposed 191–4
    history 158–9
    modelling approach 156–8, 159–60
strategies, implementation 53–4, 55–7
stroke services
    care pathways 48–9
    case study 121–6
    computerised care pathways 83–108
    follow-up 88–93
    modelling approach 125
subject gateways 42
summary of book's chapters 184–5
supportive facilitation 64
symbolic modelling, modelling approach 138
systemic approach, cf. reductionist approach 110–13, 115
Systems Architect software 133–42
    care pathway example 149–54
systems perspective, care pathways 113–14
systems view
    care pathways 109–54
    case studies 120–31

teamworking 52–3
theory of constraints (TOC) 116–17
    case study 127
training, websites 39
trials, clinical *see* clinical trials

Virtual Branch Library (VBL), heart diseases 28–31
virtual communities, websites 38

web evaluations, websites 39
websites, care pathways-related 35–9, 199–211

ZETOC 27